The International Library of Psychology

MODERN THEORIES OF THE UNCONSCIOUS

Founded by C. K. Ogden

The International Library of Psychology

GENERAL PSYCHOLOGY
In 38 Volumes

MODERN THEORIES OF THE UNCONSCIOUS

W L NORTHRIDGE

Introduction by J Laird

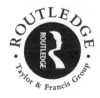

First published in 1924 by
Kegan Paul, Trench, Trubner & Co., Ltd.

Reprinted in 1999, 2001 by
Routledge

2 Park Square, Milton Park, Abingdon, Oxfordshire OX14 4RN

711 Third Avenue, New York, NY 10017

First issued in paperback 2014

Transferred to Digital Printing 2006

Routledge is an imprint of the Taylor and Francis Group, an informa company

© 1924 W L Northridge

British Library Cataloguing in Publication Data
A CIP catalogue record for this book
is available from the British Library

Modern Theories of the Unconscious
ISBN 978-0-415-21035-5 (hbk)
ISBN 978-0-415-75800-0 (pbk)
General Psychology: 38 Volumes
ISBN 978-0-415-21129-1
The International Library of Psychology: 204 Volumes
ISBN 978-0-415-19132-6

INTRODUCTION

PSYCHOLOGY seems to have reached the most interesting
stage in the development of any science—the period of
its adolescence. Compared with this, the infancy of
a science is tame, its maturity respectable and abstruse.
In the beginning, this callow creature has to collect
facts and arrange them. It allows itself pedestrian
generalisations, or else abandons science for the way-
ward premonitions of undisciplined fancy. This is
necessary, but dull, or else it is simply quaint ; and
usually it provokes only a very languid interest outside the family circle. A developed science, again, is
too assured for romance, too technical for untutored
understanding. Its theatre is an abstract firmament ;
its perplexities, filtering down to the laity, seem only
the gossip of their betters. As someone has said of the
Einstein theory : " No one but a physicist can understand
it, and the physicists never explain it."

The adolescence of a science is quite another thing ;
and if the subject at issue touches general human
interest, there is apt to be a commotion in the world.
The leaders, it is known, are guessing to some purpose,
and even the onlookers may feel themselves growing
'warm'. The furniture of ordinary experience is
rifled for analogies ; the most commonplace things
come to have an unusual appearance when they are
upset and prised open in this feverish search for clues ;
there is an air of stir and of hopefulness.

This seems to be the plight of psychology to-day,
and the 'warm' region, in the opinion both of leaders
and of onlookers, seems plainly to be the 'unconscious'. There is no question, in fact, of the promise

vii

and importance of the ideas which Mr Northridge reviews in this book.

In a sense, to be sure, psychology is one of the oldest of the sciences, but our modern psychologists think nothing of that. A few odd millennia of retarded development do not impress them. It is the last of the sciences (they tell us) to emancipate itself from theology and from metaphysics, and therefore, scientifically speaking, it is very young indeed. It was in leading-strings till the middle of the nineteenth century, and still has a tendency to return to the years of its bondage. What is more, the history of its late-born independence was dispiriting enough at the start. Escaping from one master, it was promptly annexed by another, and it spent its labour fruitlessly on a one-sided contract over the 'experimental psychology' of the special senses and of cortical localisation. This was ' science ' of a sort and therefore to be preferred to any painful, limping journey down the blind alley of introspection ; but its promise was dubious and its achievement slight.

Deliverance came from another quarter, or rather from a host of sources. Psychologists began to study the borderland of mind, abandoning for the time being what they took to be the metropolis and the citadel ; and they studied this borderland in the freest possible spirit, eliciting clues from all the sciences and from myths and legends besides. The wild mind came to instruct the tame. Spiritualism, possession, ' genius ', faith-curing, paramnesia, neurotic anomalies—these, and their like, greedily gathered, became the instruments of psychological salvation. It was the logic of the extreme case, so much more instructive than the standard mean, and the news from the borders seemed to demand a different understanding of the whole territory. The citadel was not what it seemed ; it was an emblem, not a stronghold ; a parasite of the unconscious, not its source of supplies.

INTRODUCTION

There are many, I know, who believe that this revolution in our ideas has already been gloriously accomplished. In their view, psychology has outgrown its adolescence, and the era of guesswork, on essentials, has just passed away. Ten years ago, indeed, we were guessing still, for Freud, at that time, was, comparatively speaking, unknown, and we had to conjecture, as we could, from mesmerism, or dissociated personality, or Myers's celebrated book. But now we are different, or ought to be. We are concerned to-day with the niceties, not with the foundations of the theory, and must transfer our attention to the differences within the school. We have to compare Freud with Jung or Adler, but not with their vanquished opponents ; and we need to expect to supplement their inquiries from many other sources.

This is the reason why one of M. Baudouin's reviewers finds a certain interest in one of his books. It ' indicates the path along which the Latin mind is groping towards an understanding of psycho-analysis '.

I have neither space nor inclination to argue the point in detail, but if anyone supposes that these modern conceptions of the unconscious have attained the lucidity or the mastery and economy of fundamental principles which characterise a developed science, he is most sadly mistaken. He had better go to school again, and prepare himself to answer questions in physics. This being so (and the statement could not be challenged in any competent quarter) it is plain that there is a most particular need for precisely such a book as Mr Northridge's. Unless I have misinterpreted him, Mr Northridge does in fact believe that Freud *has* worked a revolution, and that, in a general sense at least, he is very near the truth, but he also believes that we cannot afford to accept *any* such theory uncritically any more than we can afford to reject any of them dogmatically. And we are nowhere near finality in these matters, or justified in neglecting the lessons we may learn both from the mistakes and from the genius of Freud's predecessors.

I have put the point baldly and summarily; Mr Northridge goes into it in detail, and with the best possible right. He has studied his authors at first hand; he has compared them carefully and reflected on them for many years, and he has applied their views in a very extensive experience, not indeed as a professional psycho-analyst, but not the less as a serious investigator. This care, and enthusiasm, and learning give weight to his argument in detail, and there cannot be two opinions about the soundness of his general procedure.

The history of these notions, to be brief, so far from being a piece of antiquarianism, is and ought to be a thing of living interest. This is true even of the earlier stages when the word was still with the philosophers. It is also true of Myers and Janet and others like them. They also were 'warm' in their guesswork and have much to teach us. The story indeed has all the characteristics of the usual process of truth-getting, and may be compared, not unfairly, with the story of the gravitation formula before Newton, of evolution before Darwin, or of continuity before Cantor. Psychologists have still to find their Newton, even if Freud is his psychological forerunner; and therefore it is essential to review the whole of the evidence. All the sciences pursue a policy as long as it seems to pay, and the policies which are most fruitful in the end have often a shaky beginning. They are too hasty, or too crude, or lay themselves open to ruinous criticism. Therefore their interest wanes, but the stronger ideas are obscured, not destroyed, in this process. They press themselves forward once more, perhaps in an altered form, and with reference to a fresh range of facts. A series of irruptions, then, with periods of temporary defeat, and eventually a surge of converging forces—that is the history of the stronger conceptions in any science. And of such is the idea of the ' unconscious '. We are now in the surge ; it limits and constrains our guesses ; it demands clear thinking on fundamentals, and an adequate understanding of its scope and its range.

Mr Northridge knows too much of his subject to be content with any facile solution. He is anxious, instead, to help us, and has given himself to a service most urgently needed. He has shown us the principal opinions on these subjects, and the facts with which they were concerned. To neglect this course is to abandon the hope of understanding. To follow it is to invite a solution, and the invitation is very tempting in Mr Northridge's pages. For he is a critic and interpreter, as well as an annalist.

JOHN LAIRD.

PREFACE

So much has been written in recent years on the "Unconscious" that the time seems opportune to compare and contrast the various important theories that have held the field. The present book aims at a general review of this kind. The subject is "Modern Theories of the Unconscious," but as a study of current theories cannot well be entered upon without considering early theories, we include the latter in our general survey and devote the first chapter to their consideration.

On account of its importance in modern psychology, Freud's theory is kept much in evidence throughout, and frequent references are made to it when dealing with the work of other authors.

The writer takes occasion to express his especial obligation to Professor John Laird, M.A., for awakening in him an interest in the study of psychology, and in connection with the present book for many valuable criticisms and suggestions. He also gratefully acknowledges the kindness of Mr W. H. O'u. Manning, M.A., in reading the proofs.

W. L. NORTHRIDGE.

BELFAST.

CONTENTS

CONTENTS

THEORIES OF THE UNCONSCIOUS

CHAPTER I

FORMER THEORIES OF THE UNCONSCIOUS

PHILOSOPHERS did not seriously concern themselves
with the study of the unconscious earlier than the
eighteenth century. Some writers before that date give
what may be regarded as the beginning of unconscious
theory, but in none of them is a clearly defined and fully
developed doctrine to be found.

Amongst ancient philosophers, Plato and Aristotle
are of some importance for our subject. Both writers
in discussing conscious processes introduce the subject
of memory and attempt to define it. Plato, in the
Theætetus, defines it as "the preservation of a sensation." He discusses man as the subject of impressions
from without. Some of these never reach consciousness though the organism reacts to them ; some enter
consciousness and are soon forgotten, such impressions
ceasing to have any further existence ; others reach
consciousness and pass away, but are again capable of
recall. These in the interval during temporary for-
getfulness have existed in potential form, having been
retained as impressions on the soul.

Aristotle discusses the same subject in the *De Anima*.
The storing up of images, he says, is the condition of
memory. These retained images existing potentially
may be revived by association with ideas present in
consciousness.

Here in Plato and Aristotle we get an approach to the

unconscious states of the type described in modern orthodox psychology. Aristotle's theory of memory is not unlike that which Mr Bertrand Russell has developed in the *Analysis of Mind*.

There is one passage in the *Republic* of Plato * which anticipates the type of unconscious theory developed by modern psychologists in connection with the study of dreams: " Some of the unnecessary pleasures and appetites are, if I mistake not, lawful ; and these would appear to form an original part of every man ; though, in the case of some persons, under the correction of the laws and the higher appetites aided by reason, they either wholly disappear, or only a few weak ones remain ; while, in the case of others, they continue strong and numerous."

"And pray what are the appetites to which you refer?"

" I refer to those appetites which bestir themselves in sleep ; when, during the slumbers of that other part of the soul, which is rational and tamed and master of the former, the wild animal part, sated with meat or drink, becomes rampant, and pushing sleep away, endeavours to set out after the gratification of its own proper character. You know that in such moments there is nothing that it dare not do, released and delivered as it is from any sense of shame and reflection."

It is possible to find hints of unconscious theory in the works of other ancient writers, and also in early mediæval philosophy and theology, but these are not sufficiently important to detain us. Accordingly, we shall pass them by and come to the writer who may be justly credited with laying the foundations of the early theories of the unconscious, viz., Descartes. It cannot be said that Descartes made any direct contribution to the subject of the unconscious. In his writings no definite theory is set forth. His work was rather preparatory and indirect. He created those psycho-

* 571.

2

logical conditions out of which the theories to be considered in this chapter were developed. Two of these may be referred to as of great importance.

In the first place, he went much further than any of his predecessors in the emphasis he laid on consciousness and the attempt to give a full account of its contents. He held that consciousness was self-evident, that its existence could not be consistently doubted since in the effort to do so consciousness is presupposed. Further, he established a definite dualism of mind and matter. Such a separation of the psychical from the physical as this dualism involved brought into greater prominence than was previously possible the nature of the former.

It is obvious how necessary was this emphasis on the importance of consciousness as a preliminary to the development of unconscious theory. It is not likely that the unconscious could be conceived of so long as consciousness remained unexplored and obscure. Unconscious theory may, therefore, be said to have arisen in the first instance by way of contrast to consciousness when the latter, in Descartes, was fully studied.

The second consideration is that Leibniz' theory of the unconscious, which is the first of the early theories to be considered, was directly inspired by the work of Descartes.

Descartes had defined the mind as essentially " a thinking thing." According to this definition the mind thinks always. It continues to function even in conditions that suggest the contrary. " Why," Descartes asks, " is it strange that we do not remember the thoughts the soul has had when in the womb or in a stupor when we do not even remember the most of those we know when grown up in good health and awake ? For the recollection of the thoughts the mind has had during its period of union with the body it is necessary for certain traces of them to be impressed on the brain and turning and applying itself to these

3

the mind remembers. It is remarkable if the brain of an infant or one in a stupor is unfit to receive the residual impressions." *

Descartes goes further than this, and argues in accordance with his complete dualism of mind and matter that the former can perform its function without the use of the brain : " I have often shown that the mind can work independently of the brain ; for clearly there can be no use of the brain for pure intelligence, but only for imagination and sensations." †

From this position Descartes was led to classify some ideas as " innate." Such ideas are part of the original furniture of the mind and they enter consciousness as the result of the pure activity of thought   Contrasted with " innate " ideas are those called " adventitious." These depend for their origin on external conditions.

The discussion of these principles fills a large place in the work of Descartes' immediate successors. The theory of innate ideas was supported by Lord Herbert of Cherbury, and by Cudworth, but was rejected by Malebranche, who, in accordance with the doctrine of " occasionalism," declared that all ideas are impressed on the soul by God.‡ It was not, however, until the eighteenth century that, at the hands of Locke, Descartes' position received its fullest criticism.

In the *Essay*, Book II, Chapter I, these criticisms are set forth. Locke argues that " it is not more necessary for the soul always to think than for the body always to move, the perception of ideas being to the soul what motion is to the body—not its essence but one of its operations—it is quite contradictory to hold that a man can think without being sensible of it. Our being sensible of it is not necessary to any of it, but to our thoughts, and to them it is and to them it always

* Reply to Objections V.
† Reply to Objections III.
‡ Readers are referred for a full account of these discussions to Brett's *History of Psychology*, Vol. II.

4

will be necessary till we can think without being sensible of it." He goes on to urge the supporter of the theory of innate ideas to "examine his own thoughts, and thoroughly search into his understanding" and he will find that all the ideas he possesses are derived either from "the objects of his senses or the operations of his mind considered as object of his reflection." He adds that if the doctrine of innate ideas were true children and idiots would possess them, which they do not.

The discussions which we have briefly summarised furnished Leibniz with the material from the consideration of which he built up his theory of the unconscious. This theory was the answer to Locke's criticisms of Descartes' position. We are now free to consider this theory and those of subsequent German philosophers, and will then proceed to state the views of English and French philosophers on the subject.

THE UNCONSCIOUS IN GERMAN PHILOSOPHY

Leibniz

Leibniz' general philosophy supported the view that the soul always thinks, and that there are innate ideas. He represents the world as a System of Souls or monads. Each individual monad is a representation in miniature form of the whole system, but there is no communication between one monad and another. "The monads have no windows," hence no impressions reach them from outside, and knowledge has its source within the monad. In this way the theory of innate ideas received support, but not in the precise manner in which it was formulated by Descartes. Innate ideas exist NOT ACTUALLY but in LATENT or POTENTIAL FORM. They exist "as natural inclinations, dispositions and habits, and not as activities, although these powers are always accompanied by some activities often imperceptible." *

* *New Essays*, Introduction. [English Edition.]

5

Leibniz thinks that, put in this way, Locke cannot deny the truth of innate ideas. He argues that the assumption of Locke that no ideas can exist unless we are aware of them is without justification. There is a distinction to be drawn between the existence of a thing and knowledge of its existence. Bodily movements may occur of which we are not conscious. " I maintain that something goes on in the soul that corresponds to the circulation of the blood, of which we are never conscious, just as those who live near a mill do not perceive the noise it makes." *

Similarly, ideas may be in the mind of which we are not conscious. They may escape our notice, either because they are " too slight or too great in number or too even, so that they have nothing that distinguishes them clearly from one another." †

From these insensible ideas or, as Leibniz calls them, "petites perceptions" the unconscious is mainly formed. Each monad is characterised by perception and appetition in various degrees. Perception is the power of each monad to represent in itself the entire system of monads. Appetition is a name given to the striving of the monad towards completeness of representation. Three types of monad may be distinguished : First, those that relate to vegetable or plant life. In these, perception is confused and insensible, and monads at this level have applied to them the special name of " entelechies." Secondly, monads in which perception is conscious and is accompanied by memory. Animal life is typified in this class of monad. Thirdly, comes the monad that represents the human mind in which, in addition to the confused and conscious perception and memory characteristic of the lower grades of monad, we get self-consciousness or " apperception " as well.

Just as there are different grades of monad, so in the highest type there are degrees of perception ranging

* *New Essay*, p. 47.　　† *Op. cit.*, p. 47.

from those that are confused and obscure through those that are clearer and more conscious to that of self-consciousness. No definite limit to self-consciousness must be conceived. Neither is there any clear-cut division between consciousness and unconsciousness. The principle of continuity is observed throughout — self-consciousness shading off imperceptibly into consciousness and the latter into the unconscious. Thus in each monad of the highest order, or in each human mind, self-consciousness and consciousness are built up on the basis of the unconscious.

Leibniz proceeds to support this position by the argument that perception can only proceed from perception. The unconscious is, therefore, necessary to clear perception. In recovering from a state of unconsciousness, such as sleep, there must be an infinite series of perceptions through which the mind advances before clear consciousness is reached. In fact, every conscious state is a product of the unconscious in the sense that conscious states are formed out of innumerable ideas too small to be perceived separately. Thus, in attending to the roar of the sea what is heard is not the sound which each wave makes but that which is made up of all the waves together. " It must be that we are a little affected by the motion of each wave and that we have some perception of each one of these noises—small as they are—otherwise we would not have that of a hundred thousand waves ; since a hundred thousand nothings cannot make something."*
" Petites perceptions " of this kind are involved in every conscious state, and the unconscious largely consists in these. We shall now briefly state the other factor out of which, according to the Leibnizian theory, the unconscious is composed.

Monads we saw are characterised by " appetition " as well as " perception." Now, as there are various de-

* *New Essay*, p. 48.

7

grees of perception so there are of appetition. We pass from blind impulse as the lowest form of appetition through desire to volition, which is the highest. The relation between the various degrees of appetition is the same as that in perception. As there can be no clear perceptions without confused ones, so there can be no conscious striving or volition without unconscious striving or blind impulse. The vague uneasiness that we often experience, but cannot rationally account for, is the conscious effect of unconscious operations or impulses.

In two respects Leibniz' theory, as just expounded, approximates to the theory of Freud. First, in the fact that the unconscious contains more than cognitive elements ; that there is an active or conational side to it as well. The unaccountable restlessness which is so often experienced Freud explains at length as due to the operations of the unconscious. It is interesting to find the first great theory of the unconscious and the most important of the modern theories coming into close agreement on this point. At the same time it should be noted that, unlike Freud, Leibniz makes no serious attempt to answer the question, " Why do these unconscious impulses that disturb the mental equilibrium remain unconscious ? " Moreover, while Leibniz takes into account the active side of the unconscious, it is the cognitive side that is all important. Appetition on Leibniz' theory seems to depend on perception. In Freud's theory, on the other hand, as we shall see, the chief characteristic of the unconscious is its dynamical nature. The second respect in which the position of Leibniz approaches that of Freud is in the emphasis which each writer lays on the principle of determination. For Leibniz it was contrary to the law of continuity to regard absolute indeterminism as possible. " Every state of a simple substance is naturally a consequence of its preceding state in such a way that the present is big with the future and laden with the past." * One passage in particular reminds us of the Freudian psychology: " Several perceptions and inclinations conspire towards complete volition which is the result of their conflict. There are perceptions and inclinations which are individually imperceptible, but the totality of which produces an uneasiness which impels us without our seeing the ground of it." † A similar explanation is offered by Freud as a motive for individual caprice and prejudice, and many of the mistakes of everyday life that seem in themselves trivial and accidental. Mistakes of the tongue and pen are not random or chance events but are compromise formations of unconscious conflicts. Thus in both the Leibnizian and Freudian systems indeterminism is ruled out and the explanation of what seems inexplicable is sought for in the unconscious. " The error of abstract indeterminism," says Leibniz, " arises from neglect of subconscious perceptions and appetitions." Here also it is of course to be borne in mind that Freud's theory is much more thoroughly worked out than is that of Leibniz. Yet the resemblances between both theories, though general, are significant.

Kant

Kant's theory of the unconscious, as briefly stated in the *Critique of Pure Reason*, is widely different from that of Leibniz, and is in harmony with the general principles of his philosophy. A cardinal feature in his system is the view that the self is not an ultimate and unconditioned existence antecedent to and the source of experience. Consciousness of self is certainly presupposed in that of objects, but it is also true that it is only in and through consciousness of objects that our

---

* *Monadology*, section 22.
† *New Essay*, Book II., chap. i., par. 29.

9

consciousness of self becomes possible. These phases of consciousness, therefore, mutually condition each other. Self-consciousness is not in itself " noumenal " or ultimate reality. It is rather a resultant—the product of complex generative processes. There is no direct means of attaining precise knowledge of the nature of these processes. In psychological terminology they cannot be known by introspection. They are hypothetical and non-conscious. The following paragraph from Professor Norman Kemp Smith * puts the point clearly : " Now that he has shown that the consciousness of self and the consciousness of objects mutually condition each other, and that until both are attained neither is possible, he can no longer regard the mind as even possibly conscious of the activities whereby experience is brought about. The activities generative of consciousness have to be recognised themselves as falling outside it. Not even in its penumbra, through some vague form of apprehension, can they be detected."

It is not necessary to go further in order to render explicit Kant's theory. By the unconscious he meant those activities that underlie consciousness and make it possible. Kant's technical term for these is " the productive imagination." He probably introduces the term imagination in this connection because it is the creative character of imagination with which the popular mind is most familiar. " This schematism," says Kant, " is an art concealed in the depths of the soul of whose activity we are hardly ever conscious."

There is one important respect in which this theory differs from that of Leibniz. The theory of Leibniz represents the unconscious as entirely analogous to consciousness. The unconscious differs from consciousness only in accidental features of intensity and clearness. Kant, on the other hand, regards those mental processes

* *A Commentary to Kant's Critique of Pure Reason*, p. 263.

by which experience is generated as lying altogether outside consciousness. The unconscious for him does not consist in "petites perceptions," but rather in non-conscious processes.

Schopenhauer

From the Freudian point of view there is no early theory of the unconscious so important as that of Schopenhauer. His position, so far as the relative importance of the cognitive and conative factors of the unconscious is concerned, accords more fully than any of the other early theories with Freudian principles. The cognitive side of the unconscious is with him of minor importance—the will being of much greater consequence.

With regard to the unconscious on its cognitive side Schopenhauer has not much to say. He limits himself to a discussion as to how ideas appear in consciousness and disappear from it ; in other words, to a simple statement of the problem of forgetting and remembering. His account of these processes is based on the assumption that the "reality principle" in forgetting— to use the terms of modern psychology—is the only one operative in the case. The passing of ideas into the unconscious, he argues, is natural and inevitable, for we can know things only in succession. Only one idea or group of ideas can occupy consciousness at any moment ; they are succeeded by others to which they must give place, while they themselves pass into the unconscious, there to await favourable conditions of recall. "The thinking consciousness is like a magic lantern in the form of which only one thing can appear at a time, and, therefore, a distinction must be drawn between a man's knowledge and what his mind is occupied with at any moment. The former is what he knows 'potentia'; the latter is what he knows 'actu.'" *

It is the other side of his theory—that in which he considers the unconscious as consisting in conative processes or will—that is of especial interest from the standpoint of modern psychology.

His first task is to prove that the unconscious cannot wholly consist of ideas. This he endeavours to do by making plain that the recall to consciousness of unconscious ideas—a process usually explained by the law of association of ideas—can depend only in part on this principle. That this is so, the sudden emergence of unconscious material that has apparently no connection with the ideas that preceded it in consciousness proves. Some other non-cognitive factor must be present to account for this phenomenon, and Schopenhauer comes to the conclusion that the unconscious activity of the will is the factor required.

In the general philosophy of Schopenhauer the primacy of the will over cognition is recognised. The relation between will and intellect, he declares more than once, is that of the root to the fruit. The will does for our ideas what the ego, or the " I think," does for them in Kant's philosophy, i.e., it unifies and controls our thoughts. " The will as ' the thing in itself ' constitutes the inner, true, and indestructible nature of man. In itself, however, it is unconscious ; for consciousness is conditioned by the intellect, and the intellect is a mere accident of our being, for it is a function of the brain which, together with the nerves and the spinal cord connected with it, is a mere fruit, a product of the rest of the organism." †

The doctrine of the primacy of the will, though still held by some modern psychologists, calls for criticism. Such an undertaking, however, if it is to be thorough

---

* *The World as Will and Idea*, Vol. II., p. 335.
† *Op. cit.*, p. 411.

would involve a review of Schopenhauer's general philosophy which in the present connection would be irrelevant.* We will, therefore, content ourselves with saying that it is difficult to understand how the will can be altogether unconscious. It is defined by Schopenhauer as including " all wishing, shunning, hoping, fearing, loving, hating, in short all that directly concerns our weal and woe." This definition is very wide ; it includes, when precisely stated, feeling, in some at least of its forms, as well as willing, and surely these are at any rate sometimes conscious experiences. It is, however, of the essence of Schopenhauer's theory to regard the will as " the thing in itself " and, therefore, as outside the range of consciousness. Knowledge of it is only possible through its bodily " objectification."

The parallel between this theory and that of Freud is perfectly obvious. Both writers emphasise the active side of the unconscious, but more than that, both writers define this activity in the same general terms.

There is a close, though not a complete analogy between the " will " of Schopenhauer's theory and the Freudian " wish " ; the point of difference being that the latter conception is in the last analysis explained in terms of sex, while the former has a more general connotation. It includes striving of every kind.

The relation of matters sexual to the unconscious, however, has not been ignored by Schopenhauer. He discusses the possible deciding factors in the choice of a love-object, and argues that often the most potent of these are unconscious. Thus he writes : " Individuals exert a greater sexual charm the more completely they represent the idea of the race." He explains that by the " idea of the race " is meant the qualities of " beauty, nobility and grace ; " and the question of age also enters. Again he says : " That individual has the

* For a clear discussion and criticism of this point, see Professor Laird's *Problems of the Self*, p. 177.

greatest sexual charm for any other individual which, as far as possible, neutralises the other's defects by opposite defects." Schopenhauer is thinking here of the strange fact that often " the tall man prefers the short woman, the stout the thin, and the intellectual the naïve." Of these deciding factors the individual is often unconscious.

The new psychology emphasises the importance of unconscious motives in the same connection, but its explanation is entirely different from that offered by Schopenhauer. According to psycho-analysis the most potent of these unconscious factors is the resemblance of the love-object to one of the parents. The mother is held to be the first love-object of the boy, and the father of the girl, and if a man's choice in love affairs is difficult to understand, if he chooses the person that others would pronounce as most unsuitable, it is, according to psycho-analysis, because his unconscious detects in her a resemblance to his first love-object—the mother. Similarly if a member of the female sex makes love to one old enough to be her father, it is because in other respects, as well as in age, there is a resemblance between her father and her lover.

This theory seems fantastic when thus baldly stated, but it is supported in psycho-analysis by an important array of facts that cannot be easily explained away or ignored.

Herbart

Herbart's theory is characterised by a return to the more cognitive point of view of Leibniz. He takes account only of ideas and their activity. In other respects, however, his theory stands by itself.

The concept of a soul is introduced as a sort of basis for the unconscious, but it is not to be regarded either as the repository or source of ideas. It is a simple entity. Its one function is to react to ideas when these are presented to it. Like Schopenhauer, he discusses how ideas come into being in consciousness and pass away ; in other words, the problem of remembering and forgetting. It is the latter of these that chiefly concern him, and in this respect his theory approximates to the general position of Freud. There is, however, all the difference between the principles by which, according to each writer, forgetting takes place. Herbart argues that since the soul is a simple entity it is unchanging and the explanation of forgetting cannot, therefore, be found in the nature of the soul, but rather in the realm of the ideas themselves, in the principles that govern their combinations, and the tendencies that keep them apart. Ideas are driven into the unconscious according to certain mechanical principles that in form have some affinity with Freud's repression theory Both writers find forgetting due to a conflict between the ideas themselves arising out of a certain incompatibility between them, but with a radical difference in their conceptions of the nature of this incompatibility. For Freud the incompatibility is mainly one of feeling tone ; for Herbart it is purely cognitive and may be briefly stated as follows :

There are three classes of ideas or presentations—(1) Those that are alike, as for example, a sensation of blue yesterday and a sensation of blue to-day. In this case both may co-exist in consciousness. (2) Ideas that are disparate, as for example, those of sweetness and redness. These also may both remain together in consciousness. (3) Ideas that are contrary, such as those of red and green. In this case co-existence is impossible, and a conflict takes place in which the ideas strive to exclude one another. This conflict serves to transform the ideas into forces and combine them into systems. Any idea belonging to one group is aided by the whole system to which it belongs. Hence, when a new idea appears in consciousness it seeks to make

" acquaintances," for only by doing so can it hope to gain a foothold in consciousness. There are always ideas in consciousness that welcome the stranger and make him feel at home, but others will be jealous of the intruder, and will seek at once his expulsion. Whether or not the new-comer will be banished into the unconscious depends on the position and strength of the system of ideas with which it seeks attachment. On the first emergence of an idea its stay is very brief, for it has many enemies and few friends. On this account it is thrust back quickly into the unconscious. But, as in the Freudian theory, the ejected ideas do not remain in a passive position in the unconscious ; their tendency is rather to regain a foothold in consciousness. That is, as it were, the goal of their ambitions, and accordingly as they succeed or fail they are said to be " rising " or " falling." The point below which ideas become unconscious is called by Herbart " the threshold of consciousness "—a phrase which has been in common use in subsequent psychology. There are, however, two thresholds to be distinguished—the one " statical " and the other " dynamical." It is possible that in a conflict of ideas neither is capable of defeating the other. In such a case conflict need not necessarily continue. Both ideas may sink to a certain level and there co-exist without further conflict. The point in consciousness below which this is possible is called the " statical " threshold. On the other hand, ideas that are expelled altogether from consciousness are suppressed below a point called the " dynamical " threshold. Such ideas become very active, and operate as important factors in determining conscious states. The ideas below the statical threshold remain in a state of equilibrium and exercise no influence on conscious processes.

It is possible to draw a parallel between the statical and dynamical in the theory of Herbart and the fore-conscious and unconscious which the Freudian theory distinguishes; but this parallel cannot be close, since Herbart's theory only takes account of ideas and their relations, while with Freud the unconscious proper is practically non-cognitive and consists rather in conational processes. Ideas are for the most part limited to the foreconscious.

Hartmann

Hartmann's three volumes—*The Philosophy of the Unconscious*—are by far the most elaborate treatise on the unconscious during the period under review. The opening passage is worth quoting: " The sphere of consciousness is like a vine-clad hill which has been so often ploughed up in all directions that the thought of further labour has almost become loathsome to the public mind, for the looked-for treasure is never found, although rich and unexpected crops have sprung from the well-worked soil. Mankind very naturally began its researches in philosophy with the examination of what was immediately given in consciousness; may it not now be lured by the charm of novelty and the hope of a great reward, to seek the golden treasure in the mountain depths—in the noble ores of its rocky beds rather than on the surface of the fruitful earth. Undoubtedly auger and chisel and prolonged irksome labour will be needed before the golden veins are reached and, then, a tedious dressing of the ore ere the treasure be secured. Let him, however, who is not afraid of toil follow me." *

If we accept his invitation and follow him we shall be brought into unfamiliar regions, for he assigns to the unconscious a far more important rôle than any previous writer. It is even doubtful whether any writer of more recent times has attempted a more elaborate theory. The title of the work, of course, prepares us for this.

* *The Philosophy of the Unconscious*, Vol. I., pp. 1, 2.

The unconscious is worked out as a philosophy. It is an hypothesis put forth to explain a wide field of phenomena.

We shall first give a brief account of Hartmann's theory, and then show how extensively he sought to apply it. Hartmann reduces the mind to the elements of thought and will; and feeling, usually regarded by modern psychologists as a third element, is, according to him, capable of being resolved into these two. Accordingly, the unconscious is a combination of unconscious will and unconscious idea. Both conation and cognition find a place in it.

The conception of an unconscious will Hartmann found ready to hand in the philosophy of Schopenhauer; but he differs from this writer and so from the Freudian position in regarding the unconscious ideas as of equal importance. Will and idea in the unconscious are essential to each other. The latter is only potential and does not exist " realiter " until brought into being by the will. Will, on the other hand, is but an empty form until ideas are presented to it. Whether the will is conscious or not depends on whether the ideas presented to it are or are not conscious. The cognitive aspects of the unconscious are, therefore, quite as important as the conative, and the balance between these is carefully preserved throughout the entire exposition of the subject.

The bulk of Hartmann's work is devoted to the application of the unconscious, as thus defined, to a wide and varied field of phenomena. Some of these applications are reasonable enough and are such as modern psychologists are prepared to admit. Thus, he treats poetic inspiration, artistic production, sudden transition and alterations of thought as products of unconscious mentation. After referring to the experiences of Mozart and others who declare that their best thoughts came to them " in a rush " and that they were unable to give any rational account of them, he says they are " to be explained as an intrusion of the unconscious—a flash from the hidden depths of the unconscious." *

Similarly with those sudden irruptions of thought and alterations of points of view with which we are all familiar. " It regularly happens with me when I have read a work which presents new points of view essentially opposed to my previous opinions. . . . If the new ideas have made a really deep impression, they may be referred provisionally, unaccepted or undecided questions, to the court of memory, in order to be thought of again. Nevertheless the matter is only apparently laid to rest, and later when the wish or opportunity arises to give an opinion on the question we find to our great astonishment that we have undergone a mental regeneration on the point." † Hartmann calls this unconscious mental process one of digestion and assimilation, and compares it frequently with the physiological process so named.

In these and other points the findings of modern psychology are in general agreement with Hartmann's line of thought. Thus, Myers explains the facts of poetic inspiration and creative genius as due to " uprushes from the subliminal," while Wm. James' " unconscious incubation " is analogous to Hartmann's " mental assimilation."

There are, however, regions into which he, quite unwarrantably, introduces his principle, and phenomena are referred to it that are more naturally explained on other grounds. It is here that the real weakness of his theory manifests itself.

Pushed to extremes, it is made to do duty for instinct, habit, and those principles that need not be regarded as other than mechanical. Thus the migra-

* The Philosophy of the Unconscious, Vol. I., p. 279, note.
† Op. cit., p. 322.

tion of birds, and the provision by the squirrel of stores for the approaching cold are the outcome of unconscious knowledge. While in reflex action, such as stretching forth the hand to catch a piece of falling glass, and acquired dexterities, such as knitting, swimming, etc., there is evidence of design or " internal providence," which, according to Hartmann, is another name for the unconscious mind.

The climax is reached when it is suggested that " those highly purposive " movements which the stomach carries out in digestion must be presided over by unconscious intelligence. Similarly with those cases of self-healing where the mutilated parts of an organism will develop each into a separate system—or where lost parts are restored. " If there reigns in the organic healing function so wonderful a harmony, tending to a single goal, this can never be explained by the material intercommunication of the different ganglia, but only by the unity of the over-ruling principle, the unconscious." *

Few, if any, modern psychologists would think of introducing the unconscious to explain such a phenomenon, but would simply refer it either to vital or mechanical principles. To substitute the unconscious for these is to make the latter non-existent and assign to the former too wide and general a meaning.

˙THE UNCONSCIOUS IN ENGLISH PHILOSOPHY

In the section just concluded we have dealt exclusively with German writers. Our next task is to summarise the contributions to unconscious theory made by English philosophers of about the same period. A comparison of these two schools of thought reveals at once a wide difference in the attitude which each adopts towards the subject of the unconscious. German

* *The Philosophy of the Unconscious*, p. 168.

philosophers attempted to build up positive theories ; English writers concerned themselves more especially with the task of rendering explicit, and subjecting to criticism the implications of these theories. Thus, the one school may be said to be essentially positive and constructive, the other mainly negative and critical.

The problem on which the English critics of the unconscious more especially concentrated was, " How can there be unconscious ideas ? " Ideas imply consciousness, and therefore the expression " unconscious ideas," which is synonymous with unconscious consciousness, is a contradiction in terms.

Consideration of this problem led some of the English school to reject the theory altogether while others attempted so to re-state and modify it as to avoid apparent contradiction. Amongst those who adopted the former and more drastic attitude were Thomas Reid and Dugald Stewart. In the sphere of psychology Reid confined himself mainly to the task of stating and describing the conscious operations of the mind. He believed in the immediacy of consciousness which as a primary fact needed no further explanation. As for unconscious ideas, he says, " every operation of our mind is attended with consciousness, . . . and to speak of perceptions of which we are not conscious is to speak without any meaning. . . . No man can perceive an object without being conscious that he perceives it, no man can think without being conscious that he thinks."* His attitude to the unconscious is simply that it is non-existent. Dugald Stewart adopts the same negative attitude. Unlike Reid he does not regard consciousness as something for which no explanation is required. But instead of using the conception of the Unconscious he finds the doctrine of Association sufficient to account for all the facts. Ideas tend to recur in the order in which they previously occupied consciousness. Should

* *Essays on the Intellectual Powers* (1785), Vol. I., p. 264.

any link in the chain of Association be not present
in consciousness and yet an idea enters the mind that
should only come by association with this link, we are
not to suppose the latter as unconsciously existing.
What has happened is rather that it made a momentary
appearance in consciousness, and passed away so
swiftly that it was impossible for consciousness to be
aware of its presence. Ideas in which we are especially
interested, he holds, are more easily retained in, and
recalled to consciousness than others " that do not
arouse our curiosity." In this part of his theory there
are many suggestions of the Freudian view, which makes
forgetting depend on the painfulness of ideas and
remembering on their pleasurable " affect." " Those
objects are easily remembered which affect any of our
passions." *

The majority of the English school attempted to
re-state the principle of the unconscious rather than
deny it, and three different lines of modification may
be distinguished. The first of these we owe to Sir Wm.
Hamilton, whose treatment of the subject is more
exhaustive than any other English writer of this period.

Instead of regarding the unconscious as consisting of
" unconscious ideas," "presentations," etc., he prefers to
speak of " mental modifications " or " mental latency."

There are three types of mental latency:

1. The knowledge which each person possesses far
exceeds that of which he is aware at any moment.
Such mental possessions are at our disposal when we
need them, but while absent from consciousness they
exist in a latent form. " The infinitely greater part
of our spiritual treasure lies always beyond the sphere
of consciousness, hid in the obscure recesses of the
mind." †

2. There are " systems of knowledge " and " possi-

* *The Philosophy of the Human Mind*, p. 216.
† *Metaphysics*, chap. xviii.

bilities of action " of which we are entirely unconscious in normal waking life, but which reveal themselves in delirium, somnambulism, and other abnormal states. Coleridge's famous story is introduced to illustrate this type or level of unconsciousness. An illiterate young woman was stricken with fever and in her delirium began fluently to recite Greek, Latin, and Hebrew sentences. Her past history was traced step by step by those whose interest in the case was awakened, and it was discovered that in early life she had lived for some time in the home of a Rabbi whose habit it had been to read aloud from Greek, Latin, and Hebrew writings. The conclusion reached by those who investigated the case was that the impressions made in those early days had persisted throughout the years, and now in her delirium when the "Surface" consciousness was removed they became active, and the sentences that she heard, but did not understand, were reproduced.

3. There are mental modifications, of which we are unconscious, but which are constantly influencing our conscious life, and upon which consciousness depends. At this point his theory coincides with that of Leibniz, though he avoids the precise expressions in which the theory of the latter is couched. "When we look at a distant forest we perceive a certain expanse of green. Now the expanse of which we are conscious is evidently made up of parts of which we are not conscious, the greenness of the forest is made up of the greenness of the leaves, that is, the total impression of which we are conscious is made up of an infinitude of smaller impressions of which we are not conscious."

There follows a criticism of Dugald Stewart's negative attitude towards unconscious theory, in which it is asserted that nothing can consistently be said to enter consciousness of which there is no memory, "If there be no memory there can be no consciousness." * If

* *Metaphysics*, p. 355.

A calls up C, although there is no direct connection between them, it must be because of a middle term B which is a mental modification existing unconsciously.

In J. S. Mill and Dr Wm. Carpenter we have a modification of the theory of the unconscious along a different line. Hamilton's statement of the subject is unacceptable to Mill, since he finds the notion of " unconscious mental modifications " quite as contradictory as that of " unconscious ideas." Hence, he prefers to speak of " nervous modifications " rather than " mental modifications ; " that is, he reduces the idea of the unconscious to a physiological concept. " The essential part of the phenomena is that we have or once had many sensations, and that many sensations do or once did enter into our train of thought, which sensations and ideas we afterwards, in the words of James Mill, are under an acquired capacity of attending to . . . we know that these lost ideas leave traces of having existed, they continue to be operative in introducing other ideas by association . . . they exist in the shape of unconscious modifications of nerves." *

Dr Wm. Carpenter in his *Mental Physiology* works out this point of view more fully in his theory of " Unconscious Cerebration." He thinks that such a method of defining the unconscious is not open to the charge brought against the various statements of the theory by the German school—or by Sir Wm. Hamilton—for it is not a psychological or philosophical, but a physiological theory. " Since in the systems of philosophy long prevalent in this country consciousness has been almost uniformly taken as the basis of all strictly mental activity, it seems convenient to designate as functions of the nervous system all those operations which lie below that level, and there is this advantage in approaching the subject from the physiological side that the study of the automatic action of other

* *Examination of Sir Wm. Hamilton's Philosophy*, pp. 354-355, 3rd edition.

24

parts of the nervous system furnishes a clue by the guidance of which we may be led to the scientific elucidation of many phenomena that would otherwise remain obscure and meaningless." *

There is yet a third type of approach to the subject of the unconscious which is illustrated in MacNish's *Philosophy of Sleep* and Abercrombie's *Intellectual Powers*. These writers discuss at considerable length the subject of dreams, delirium, somnambulism, and kindred phenomena of the type dealt with so fully in modern psychology. While these writers do not attempt to relate these phenomena to any definite theory of unconsciousness, yet they anticipate, in some measure, the work of later psychologists, such as Pierre Janet, in introducing the conception of a contraction or splitting of consciousness, as an hypothesis to account for the abnormal in mental life. In this way the apparent awkwardness and contradiction of the theories of unconsciousness presented in German philosophy have been avoided.

To sum up this section, the English writers approach the subject of the unconscious mainly from a critical point of view ; they either adopt an entirely negative attitude toward it, or else concern themselves with the attempt so to re-state the theory as to make it more acceptable to reason. This latter procedure has resulted in the modification of unconscious theory in the forms in which it was expounded by the German school, and three methods of modification may be distinguished: (1) That of Sir Wm. Hamilton who substitutes unconscious " mental modifications " for unconscious ideas; (2) That of J. S. Mill and Dr Wm. Carpenter who lean toward a purely physiological theory ; (3) That of MacNish and Abercrombie who avoid the word " unconscious " altogether and speak instead of " contraction of consciousness."

* *Mental Physiology*, pp. 316-317.

THEORIES OF THE UNCONSCIOUS

THE UNCONSCIOUS IN FRENCH PHILOSOPHY

Our account of early theories of the unconscious would scarcely be complete without some reference to the subject as treated in French philosophy. It is notable that while the early theories had their real origin in the work of a French writer (Descartes), yet the subject of the unconscious is largely ignored in the French philosophy of the eighteenth century. The explanation of this is to be found in the fact that French philosophy of this period drew its inspiration largely from the English Empirical School, of which Locke was a leading representative. Voltaire had become, after his visit to England, a great admirer of Locke, but there is nothing in his writings that is important as a contribution to psychology. Diderot wrote on the life of a blind man and in this novel way considered the mental experiences of a man deprived of one sense. His work was regarded as a contribution to individual psychology. But his empirical method did not lend itself to the development of unconscious theory.

Condillac was one of the most important of the French empiricists. He was a close student of Locke, but instead of beginning with sensation and reflection as independent sources of knowledge, he held that sensation was prior to, and the basis of reflection. He presents his theory in a picturesque way by imagining a statue possessed with only one sense, that of smell, through which impressions reach the soul. The first sensation entirely occupies the mind ; it is the sole content of consciousness. But on the arrival of a new sensation one of two possibilities is open : either the two remain together in the mind, and the power of comparison is brought into being, or the second sensation throws the first back, and then we have the foundation of Memory, since it is possible to bring the lost sensations back again to consciousness.

Cabanis was a pupil of Condillac. He worked out more fully the theory of his master, his chief contribution being the introduction of physiological factors as the basis of conscious states. Condillac's theory was deficient here, and he had to fall back on a form of occasionalism as the ultimate explanation of the origin of ideas. Cabanis held that what determined the quality of consciousness was the whole state of the organism, and so he at once dismissed as unnecessary the doctrine of Occasionalism.

When we pass to the nineteenth century we find French thought in revolt against the materialism of Cabanis. Writers such as Royer-Collard, Cousin, Jouffroy, and Maine de Biran, represent a complete reaction from this point of view. These men criticised the work of their predecessors because of its failure to account for the perceptions of beauty, moral truth, and so forth, as well as on the ground that it did not take into account the will. The result was the development of a theory of activity which led to an aggressive voluntaryism, and a reaction towards a spiritualistic psychology. Notwithstanding this reversal from the position of the materialists there is scarcely anything in the writings of this group, that is of interest to the student of the unconscious. Biran may be linked up with Leibniz because of his insistence on activity, and also because of the fact that he recognises certain distinct levels in consciousness. He speaks of the affective, the sensitive, the perceptive, and the reflective consciousness.

The first of these is common to both man and animal and it is described as a form of consciousness that is obscure and without self-recognition. The sensitive and perceptive levels stand for a higher stage of complexity and clearness, and so on until the highest form of consciousness is reached in reflective thought or self-consciousness.

The work of Ribot inaugurates a new era in France so far as psychology is concerned. The Materialistic school was followed by that of the Spiritualists, but with Ribot may be said to begin a new development—that of French experimental psychology. Ribot himself has little to say with regard to the unconscious. He discusses in his review of English and German psychology the theory of "Unconscious Cerebration" and other current theories, but he adopts on the whole a non-committal attitude. "Unconscious Cerebration" cannot satisfactorily explain "the series of adaptations, corrections, and rational operations" that are involved in the creative imagination. On the other hand, the psychological theories in vogue involve "the belief that if we descend from clear to obscure consciousness, and from this to unconsciousness that manifests itself in motor reaction, the first state, thus successfully impoverished, still remains down to its lowest term identical in basis with consciousness." * While, however, Ribot leaves us with no definite theory of the unconscious he recognises that some theory is necessary to explain the facts of the mental life.

More important is the fact that he was called to the first chair of French Experimental and Comparative Psychology,† and that he was interested in the subject of pathology. In this way began the movement with which we associate the names of Charcot, Pierre Janet, and others whose work from the standpoint of the unconscious is of great importance. The work of these writers, however, is to be included in the modern theories proper, and it will be considered in Chapter III.

* *The Creative Imagination*, p. 341.
† See Brett, *A History of Psychology*, Vol. III., p. 249.

CHAPTER II

WE shall begin our exposition of the modern theories with an account of Myers' " Subliminal Self." This is appropriate, not only because in point of time it comes earlier than most of the modern theories, but also because it stands alone, both as regards the phenomena which it is intended to explain and the form in which it is presented.

The phenomena in which Myers was especially interested are generally known as " psychical." They came under his notice as a member of the Society for Psychical Research. It was for the purpose of investigating in a scientific way certain extraordinary phenomena, hitherto regarded as either illusory or supernatural, that this Society came into existence. Whether the phenomena in question were interpreted one way or the other depended largely on factors of temperament and training. Writers of the time, such as Barrett, Myers, and Sidgwick, who were the leaders of the newly-formed Society, were not prepared beforehand to accept either of the current explanations. They approached the phenomena with open minds, decided to deal with them in a scientific way, and thus find out what their real interpretation might be. In the course of the Society's experiments and investigations much fraud and deception were discovered, many of the so-called supernatural occurrences being traced to ingenious human trickery. There was, however, a residue of phenomena that could not be accounted for in this way. For these a threefold principle of explanation was adopted, the subliminal self, telepathy, and spiritualism. Many of the phenomena were accounted for by the first of these alone, but for the more complicated cases it was found necessary to fall back on telepathy and spirit communication. These, however, it was discovered, operated through the subliminal self, and not directly on the upper, or surface consciousness. The subliminal self became, therefore, the main principle in Myers' psychology. Some of the phenomena were wholly explained by it, others only partially, but in practically every case the subliminal was involved.

The conception of the unconscious which Myers offers is quite as peculiar as the phenomena dealt with, and on this account also his theory demands separate treatment. In the following passage, which we quote from the introduction to *Human Personality*, the main features of his theory are presented : " The word subliminal has already been used to define those sensations which are too feeble to be individually recognised. I propose to extend the meaning of the term, so as to make it cover all that takes place beneath the ordinary threshold, or say, if preferred, outside the ordinary margin of consciousness—not only those faint stimulations whose very faintness keeps them submerged, but much else which psychology as yet scarcely recognises ; sensations, thoughts, emotions, which may be strong, definite, and independent, but which by the original constitution of our being seldom emerge into that supra-liminal current of consciousness which we habitually identify with ourselves. Perceiving that these submerged thoughts and emotions possess the characteristics which we associate with conscious life I feel bound to speak of a *subliminal* or *ultra-marginal* consciousness— a consciousness which we shall see, for instance, uttering or writing sentences quite as complex and coherent as the supraliminal consciousness could make them. Perceiving further that this conscious life beneath the threshold, or beyond the margin, seems to be no discontinuous or intermittent thing ; that not only are these isolated subliminal processes comparable with isolated supraliminal processes, but that there also is a continuous subliminal chain of memory involving just that kind of individual and persistent revival of old impressions and response to new ones, which we commonly call a self—I find it permissible to speak of subliminal selves, or more briefly of a subliminal self. I do not intend by using this term to assume that there are two correlative and parallel selves existing always within each of us. Rather, I mean by the subliminal self that part of the self which is commonly subliminal ; and I conceive that there may be not only co-operations between these quasi-independent trains of thought but also upheavals and alternations of personality of many kinds so that what was once below the surface may, for a time, or permanently rise above it. And I conceive also that no self of which we can here have cognisance is in reality more than a fragment of a larger self revealed in a fashion at once shifting and limited through an organism not so framed as to afford it full manifestation.''

This theory differs widely from those considered in the preceding chapter. The early theories are largely bound up with the philosophical presupposition of their authors. On this account they may generally be described as a priori. All the modern theories, on the other hand, have been built up out of a close study of mental data, and, for the most part, the aim of their authors is practical. The theories are meant to be clues to and explanations of obscure mental phenomena, and unusual behaviour. Some psycho-analysts put the theory of Myers in the same category as those we have considered, on account of certain supposed philosophical implications which it contains, but the method of Myers was quite as scientific as those which the medical school of psychologists employed, though his results are widely different from theirs.

Myers also himself, in the passage we have quoted, claims at once for his theory important advances on those of the early writers. The subliminal, he says, "contains not only those faint stimulations whose faintness keeps them submerged, but much else, which psychology has scarcely yet recognised—sensations, thoughts, emotions, which may be strong, definite and independent."

This claim is borne out by Professor James in his chapter on Myers in his *Memories and Studies*. "I cannot but think," he says, "that the most important step forward that has occurred in psychology since I have been a student of that science is the discovery, first made in 1886, that in certain subjects at least, there is not only the consciousness of the ordinary field with its usual centre and margin but an addition thereto in the shape of a set of memories, thoughts, and feelings which are extra-marginal and outside of the primary consciousness altogether, but yet must be classed as conscious facts of some sort able to reveal their presence by unmistakable signs."

Our review of the earlier writers at once reveals that both Myers and Professor James are here claiming too much. We found, especially in the theories of Leibniz and Schopenhauer, much more than " stimulations " too faint to enter consciousness. So far as this point is concerned we are only dealing with differences of degree between Myers' theory and those of his predecessors. The more radical differences will become apparent as we proceed.

One point in the exposition of Myers' theory in the light of its application throughout the book strikes us as very important ; there seem to be two sides to his theory—two distinct aspects to the subliminal self. Myers himself did not render this fact very clear, with the result that confusion is inevitable where the point is not grasped.

His theory in one form means very little more than the unconscious in orthodox psychology. It consists of those mental elements that are " too weak to rise into direct notice," together with certain elements that are extra-marginal. On the other hand, he uses the same term, " the subliminal," for something not recognised in orthodox psychology—a " profound faculty," the intuitions of which are submerged, not by their own weakness, but by the constitution of man's personality. The word " soul " is used synonymously with the subliminal in this sense. Thus in the opening passage of Chapter II we are told that every organism is ruled and unified by a " soul or spirit absolutely beyond our present analysis—a soul which has originated in a spiritual or 'metetherial' environment, which, while embodied, subsists in that environment and which will still subsist therein after the body's decay." Another synonym in constant use throughout the book is " subliminal " or " supernal faculty."

Thus there are distinguished in his theory two forms of the subliminal : the subliminal as a region of the mind built up in the course of individual experience ; and that " profounder faculty " or " soul " which inhabits a metetherial environment.

It is fairly plain that in dealing with the wide and varied field of phenomena reviewed in *Human Personality* the author applies to some the subliminal, in the first sense, and to others that in the second. Henceforth, for the sake of convenience, we shall distinguish these forms of the theory by the terms Subliminal I. and Subliminal II.

In the chapter on Disintegrations of Personality only

Subliminal I. is made use of as far as we can judge. The subliminal in this sense is described as having been formed by the agency of an idea or group of ideas that become separated from the main stream of conscious- ness. These may form " a new parasitic centre " and draw to themselves so many psychic elements that they develop into a sort of secondary personality. He goes on to tell us that we cannot understand the puzzles of hysteria unless " we keep our eyes fixed upon a thres- hold of ordinary consciousness above which certain perceptions and faculties ought to be but are not always maintained and upon a ' hypnotic stratum ' or ' region of the personality to which hypnotic suggestion appeals ' and include faculty and perception which surpass the supraliminal but whose operations are capricious and dream-like, inasmuch as they are, so to say, in a debat- able region between two rules—the known rule of the supraliminal self and the conjectural rule of a fuller and profounder self rarely reached by any artifice that our present skill suggests." *

In this passage not only are the two forms of the subliminal recognised but their relative positions are indicated.

Myers next turns to the subject of genius, and here it would seem he makes use of the two forms of the subliminal. Genius is defined as " the power of utilising a wider range than other men can utilise of faculties in some degree innate in all—a power of appropriating the results of subliminal mentation to subserve the supraliminal stream of thought. . . . An ' Inspiration of Genius ' will be in truth a subliminal uprush, an emergence into the current of ideas which the man is consciously manipulating of other ideas which he has not consciously originated, but which have shaped themselves in profounder regions of his being." † This definition is quite general, but in the argument that

* *Op. cit.*, Vol. I., p. 43.   † *Op. cit.*, Vol. I., p. 71.

follows various degrees of genius are distinguished. Some of these are explained, it would seem, by Subliminal I., others by Subliminal II.

Thus, he says, dealing with some of its manifestations, such as the sudden exercise of unsuspected strength and skill in great emergencies, we are aware not only of conscious ideas but "also of a substratum of fragmentary, automatic, liminal ideas, of which we take small account. These are bubbles that break on the surface ; but every now and then there is a stir among them. There is a rush upwards as of a subaqueous spring ; an inspiration flashes into the mind for which our conscious effort has not prepared us." * So far as our judgment goes there is involved in this statement little more than would be admitted by the majority of psychologists to-day.

When, however, Myers comes to deal with those higher degrees of genius manifested in the "computative gift" of "calculating boys" who are "capable of performing 'on their heads,' and almost instantaneously, problems for which ordinary workers would require pencil and paper and a much longer time," the supernal faculty or Subliminal II. is introduced. The founders of religions and some traditional saints are also cited as instances of genius of this high order. "The monitions of the Dæmon of Socrates . . . did convey to that great philosopher precisely the kind of telæsthetic or precognitive information which forms the sensitive's privilege to-day."

The same double aspect of his theory may be traced in the discussion on sleep. "I think," he says, "that there is evidence to show that many facts or pictures which have never even for a moment come within the apprehension of the supraliminal consciousness are nevertheless retained by the subliminal memory, and are occasionally presented in dreams with what seems a

* *Op. cit.*, Vol. I., p. 77.

definite purpose." This and other passages, which one might quote, show that some of the phenomena of sleep are regarded by Myers as due to the Subliminal I. But on approaching the consideration of more striking phenomena, he significantly says: "Thus far, indeed, the sleep faculties which we have been considering, however strangely intensified, have belonged to the same class as the normal faculties of waking life. We have now to consider whether we can detect in sleep any manifestation of supernormal faculty. We shall find, I think, that there are coincidences of dreams with truth which neither pure chance nor any subconscious mentation of an ordinary kind will adequately explain." * There follow instances of dreams of a "supernormal" kind, and a discussion of the subjects of telæsthesia or "sensation at a distance" and telepathy or thought transference. Knowledge of important events which are first made known in dreams, he thinks, cannot be explained without telæsthesia and telepathy. The latter of these operates through Subliminal II., in which the transmitted messages often remain latent until suitable conditions prevail for their emergence into consciousness. The former is treated as a characteristic of the same faculty.

In the chapter on Hypnotism much that we associate with the work of Coué is anticipated ; as when he argues that suggestion by the hypnotiser is of little service until the subject receives it and makes it his own. Hetero-suggestion must become auto-suggestion. But this is not enough. The subliminal must come into play. Suggestion is "a successful appeal to the subliminal self." Here again it is easy to distinguish his use of the two forms of the subliminal. He tells us that the subliminal self, to which successful appeal is made, "is not necessarily the self in its most central, most unitary aspect, but to some one at least of those

* *Op. cit.*, Vol. I., p. 135.

strata of subliminal faculty which I have in an earlier chapter described." *   He further explains that hypnotism offers an opportunity for experimentally raising " subliminal mentation." Now, if it is the supernal faculty alone he has in mind in dealing with the phenomena of hypnotism rather ludicrous results follow, for he cites those cases where, at the suggestion of the hypnotiser the subject takes vinegar for wine, sees a dog where there is no dog, or believes himself to be someone else. If suggestion consists in raising the thoughts of the subliminal self into supraliminal consciousness, then we must suppose that the subliminal possesses these strange experiences and that suggestion simply brings them above the threshold. This is obviated if we suppose the subliminal in its more simple form to be involved. All that happens in this case is that the idea suggested by the hypnotiser works itself out when competing ideas are absent and the critical faculties are in abeyance.

In other hypnotic experiences, however, in which moral and physical cures are effected, and in which hypnosis is " telepathically produced at a distance " and " travelling clairvoyance " takes place, the supernal faculty is introduced definitely. These cures, he argues, can only be explained by assuming some energy " indrawn " from the " metetherial environment " in which this faculty has its home.

The teaching of the New Nancy School, of which some account will be given in the next chapter, has made it clear that no such conception is necessary in the case of cures wrought by suggestion. Once ideas of health become lodged in the mind and are not interfered with by opposing ones, they tend to realise themselves. The questions of telepathy and " travelling clairvoyance " both belong to those phenomena called " psychical " with which Myers particularly deals towards the end

* *Op. cit.*, Vol. I., p. 169.

of his work, and in connection with which the supernal faculty plays an important rôle. When we reach this part of Myers' teaching Subliminal I. is of little use, the supernal faculty or Subliminal II. is everything.

Let us briefly indicate how this principle is applied by Myers to so-called " psychical " phenomena.

Already we have indicated how, according to Myers, telepathy requires for the explanation of delayed messages the hypothesis of a supernormal faculty. " Travelling clairvoyance," which is really, as stated by Myers, a form of telepathy—a method of gaining knowledge of places and events beyond the range of the ordinary sensory powers, involves the same faculty. In the phenomena of " travelling clairvoyance," he says, " there is a fusion of all our powers of supernormal faculty, the subliminal self exercises its farthest-reaching supernormal powers."

From a consideration of these " self projections " of " spirits still in the flesh," Myers easily passes to an inquiry regarding the agency of disincarnate spirits who communicate with those still on earth. It is not certain whether all such communications are actually from disincarnate spirits. It is possible that many of them may have been transmitted telepathically before the death of the agent took place, and may have remained latent in the subliminal of the recipient until suitable conditions were present for their emergence into the supraliminal consciousness. But this explanation is not quite so plausible in those cases in which messages reach the subject long after the death of the agent. It can scarcely be supposed that they could remain latent for years. Neither is this explanation satisfactory in many of the phenomena of " table tilting," " table wrapping," " planchette writing," etc. ; some messages, that in these and other ways are automatically written, may emanate from the automatist's subliminal, even though he may be ignorant of ever possessing the particular information which the messages disclose ; or they may originate in the minds of others and be conveyed telepathically to the sub-liminal of the automatist, and then be communicated to the supraliminal consciousness. But Myers and other members of the Society for Psychical Research have recorded well-authenticated instances that do not seem at all amenable to these principles of explanation. Messages are rapped out or written out that could not have been present subliminally or supraliminally in any mind still on earth : such at any rate is the con-tention of Myers. For the explanation of such cases he introduces the " spiritualistic hypothesis " in which it is held that the organism may be invaded and con-trolled for a time by a disembodied spirit—the per-sonality who generally inhabits it disappearing during that period. Here there is no question either of telepathy or subliminal faculty, the communicating spirit simply taking control of the agent's brain and nervous system and transmitting its communications in this way.

There is, however, another form of the spiritualistic hypothesis according to which information about the spiritual world is derived by the excursion thereto of the spirit during the trance state, or by telepathetic intercourse between Subliminal II. of the " sensitive " and a disembodied spirit. In the passage in which this aspect of the theory is stated the " subliminal self " is actually identified with the " incarnate spirit."

Since it is no part of our task to estimate the value of the spiritualistic hypothesis, or to consider the cogency of the arguments in support of it, we will pass over the instances that Myers records. Readers may examine them for themselves. Our only concern is with the conception of the subliminal which, as we have seen, is made so much of in the elucidation of these and kindred phenomena. We have stated briefly the position of Myers, and have expressed the view that two forms of the Subliminal Self are to be recognised ; now one form and now the other is made use of according to the nature of the phenomena dealt with. It remains for us to state two considerations that in our judgment tell against the general acceptance and value of Myers' theory.

In the first place, the value of the theory must be estimated in the light of its aim. The main purpose of the hypothesis is definitely stated by its author. As already indicated Myers' chief concern was the scientific explanation of " psychical " phenomena. He saw that there was no possibility of this unless " psychical " phenomena could be co-ordinated with psychological phenomena of the kind already recognised as capable of being submitted to the ordinary tests of science. His theory of the subliminal self was introduced for this purpose. This hypothesis must, therefore, be viewed principally as a unifying and co-ordinating agency and if it fails in this respect the greater part of its value is gone.

Now, our interpretation of Myers' theory is either correct or not correct. If the former then he has failed in his main task. For if for one set of phenomena the subliminal in one sense is used, and for another the subliminal in a different sense, then the co-ordination of the phenomena reviewed has not been achieved. There are two principles at work instead of one.

If, on the other hand, we are to recognise only one form of the subliminal, then its statement is hopelessly confusing, for now it is put in terms of orthodox psychology and again in more mystical terms as inhabiting " a metetherial environment," etc. Further, if this is the interpretation intended still co-ordination is not attained in any but a verbal sense, for the Subliminal II. seems inappropriate when applied to some of the phenomena discussed.   It is very unlikely that Myers himself would have introduced such a conception if his investigations were confined to the type of phenomena considered in the early chapters of his book.   He was led to adopt it in view of the supernormal phenomena, the explanation of which was his chief concern, and because he desired the co-ordination of these with the more normal types of phenomena.   A theory, however, that may be necessary in dealing with the former may not be appropriate or adequate as an explanation of the latter.   The fact is that Myers' theory is too simple to unify and explain the great variety of phenomena reviewed and so he has to introduce by the side of the Subliminal Self other conceptions of an auxiliary kind. No matter how we interpret the theory of Myers, therefore, the co-ordination of abnormal with normal phenomena at which he aimed has not been accomplished.

The question is whether the newer theories of the unconscious that are at hand may not bring about the result which Myers hoped for, and, at the same time, enable us to dispense with telepathy and spiritism.

If this is at all likely, then, the theory of the Subliminal Self must be displaced by these.   We cannot here expound the theories of the unconscious which we owe to modern analytical psychology, but in so far as these theories throw light on " psychical " phenomena they may be referred to.

The principle of dissociation of personality, which we owe to the researches of Pierre Janet, has explained much that formerly was obscure in psycho-pathology. It is only quite recently, however, that this principle has begun to be applied in the field of " psychical " research.   Though the workers in this field express their views tentatively, and ask us to proceed cautiously, yet the results so far obtained are encouraging.   One thing may be stated quite definitely, the mechanism in the " mediumistic " trance is identical with that of the hypnotic state and with that of certain forms of hysteria.

Some of the secondary personalities that result from dissociation of the primary self are, as we shall see in the next chapter, of the co-conscious type, *i.e.*, if A has a secondary personality B, then while A may know nothing of B, B may know everything of A. B in this case is to be identified with " the control " in the mediumistic trance. The strangeness of the knowledge which B imparts in the trance, and which is attributed to a supernormal agency, is thus accounted for by medical psychology.

In his book, *The Naturalisation of the Supernatural*, Mr Podmore tells us that most of the so-called spiritual-istic phenomena can be explained by this principle of dissociation. Loss of personal identity through dissociation happens, he says, " not only in the more extreme pathologic cases, but even in profound hypnotism or in the spontaneous trance observed at spiritualistic séances. Even the talking table will personify itself, and the hand of the automatic writer will frequently proclaim its separate individuality. The new consciousness will then speak of the normal personality, as ' he ' or ' she ' or the ' medium ' and give to itself a wonderful new name. The name chosen will be apt to reflect the wishes of the entranced subject, or the prepossession of the bystanders ; it may be that of a Hebrew prophet, one of Solomon's genii, an Indian chief, or a deceased friend of those present " (p. 284).

Notwithstanding this, Podmore had to admit that psycho-pathology did not account for all the occurrences that had been investigated by the Society for Psychical Research. Knowledge has been imparted in the trance state during the séance that could not be traced to any natural source.

The question remains whether the more recent

developments in the field of psycho-pathology have brought us any nearer to a natural explanation of this supernormally acquired knowledge.

The work of psycho-analysts has afforded a better understanding of the meaning of dissociation than was previously available, and it is in this direction we must look for the further elucidation of psychical phenomena. A central point in the teaching of psycho-analysts is that dissociation is brought about by the general tendency to thrust the painful—because it *is* painful — out of consciousness. Dr Mitchell, in his recent book, *Medical Psychology and Psychical Research*, has complained that so far the principles of psycho-analysts have not been applied to the phenomena of dual or multiple personality, and he attempts such an application himself. Amongst the various cases of multiple personality described by him the most is made of that of Doris Fitscher. The story of this case has been recorded at great length by Dr Walter Prince and Dr Hyslop in the American *Proceedings of the Society for Psychical Research*. In the course of his investigations of this case Dr Prince discovered in Doris no fewer than five distinct personalities. The first was Sick Doris, who was always depressed and careworn, the second was Margaret, who though lovable was often mischievous and malicious, and frequently had her revenge on Sick Doris if the latter in any way displeased her. During a scene in which Sick Doris in her sleep was being maltreated Margaret, the third and most important personality, was discovered. Dr Prince had been remonstrating with Margaret about her ill-treatment of Sick Doris, but without success. Then he attempted to take away her power by suggestion—" Attempting suggestion I began to say impressively ' I am going to take away your power. You are growing weaker. You are losing your strength '. The struggles became weaker.

43

Finally I said 'Your strength is gone. You are powerless'. All striving ceased, the face changed, and she (S. D.) awoke. She now appeared extremely languid and spoke with difficulty, but said that she felt no pain. Her vital forces seemed to be ebbing away and she gradually passed into a condition which made Mrs Prince and me think, not for the first time, that she was dying. Her pulse descended to 54, and became feeble. She seemed only half-conscious, but occasionally looked wonderingly at the two who were sitting by her, affected by their impression that she was near her end. At length she murmured : 'Am I dying ? ' (I think so.) 'Don't you want to go ? ' She smiled peacefully, as though both glad to go and to know that she was to be missed. She looked singularly unlike her afternoon self, the very shape of her face altered—it seemed thinner, as though she had passed through a period of sickness since. Under the spell of considerable emotion I was looking into her eyes, and presently her gaze fixed upon mine, and with parted lips she continued to look, not rigidly, but dreamily and peacefully, while we waited for the end which we thought so near. After some time it suddenly struck me that her gaze and feature were unnaturally fixed— I stooped to examine her.

" Just then a voice issued from her lips, though no other feature moved : 'You must get her out of this. She is in danger.' It was as startling as lightning from the blue sky. Of course I thought it must be Margaret speaking, but there was a calm authority in her tone which was new. I shook the girl gently, her face did not change. 'Shake her harder,' the voice went on. 'Hurry ! Hurry ! ' It was evident that Doris was in a profound state of hypnosis, and I began vigorous measures to bring her out, with the result that her eyes rolled and her limbs moved. Shaking her and shouting in her ear brought her to a sitting position. 'Walk

44

her ! walk her ! ' said the voice. At first there was difficulty in carrying out this order, she stumbled and tended every moment to collapse upon the carpet. Directions occasionally continued to issue from the lips . . . directions which I never thought of disregarding, they were delivered with such authority and characterised by such good sense. Finally we heard, ' She is coming to herself now ; she will be all right soon.' No more directions were given, and almost at once the face showed more animation and intelligence."*

Sleeping Margaret came at length to be identified by Dr Prince, chiefly under the influence of Dr Hyslop who was an extreme spiritualist, with a spirit, and certain purported supernormal occurrences were attributed to her. Dr Mitchell, however, pointed out that the evidence for this is far from convincing, and that there is no reason to suppose that the voice of sleeping Margaret " had any other source than some deeper stratum of her own being. This deeper and more sane personality, recognising that Dr Prince had lost his bearing, feels the need to take control herself " (pp. 172-173). Sleeping Margaret was asked by Dr Prince whether she was a spirit. This she at first denied, but later on admitted. The fact that Dr Hyslop had so much to do with the case, however, suggests that she was induced to make this confession.

A study of the history of Doris reveals that at the age of three she was taken from the arms of her mother by her father during a drunken quarrel and dashed on the floor. To the shock which on this occasion was experienced may be traced the origin of the disintegration of her personality. From the age of three to that of seventeen three personalities existed side by side, "Real " Doris and Margaret as alternating personalities, and sleeping Margaret as a co-conscious personality.

At the age of seventeen her mother, whom she adored,

* *Medical Psychology and Psychical Research*, pp. 170-172.

died. Doris "managed to retain her individuality until she had performed the last offices in her power for her dead idol, whereupon Margaret took her place. Almost immediately thereafter a terrible pain shot through the left cerebral hemisphere, then vanished, and a new personality, afterwards to be known as Sick Doris, came into the drama." * Sick Doris is described on her first appearance as an " infantile personality." She lost all memory of what Doris or Margaret had learnt. She knew no one and could not speak ; all affection and all grief disappeared, and " she was as one born with an adult body."

There is much in this story that psycho-analysis helps us to interpret. Freud explains all cases of dissociation as due to the repression of unpleasant ideas, or the attempt to escape from a painful situation. Evidently the disappearance of the Real Doris and the emergence of a new personality were " protective reactions " against a situation that had become unbearable. Whether the painful in the precise sense in which Freud defines it as the motive of repression were present, we cannot tell, for so far as we know the case was not " analysed." But the general idea of a flight into sickness, which is the explanation of many cases of neurosis, seems applicable in this case.

Taking all this into account, while Dr Mitchell is not dogmatic yet he leans to the view that Sleeping Margaret is not a spirit but a co-conscious personality that has been brought into existence by the mechanism of dissociation.

Freud himself has recently entered the field of " psychical " phenomena and has sought to relate them to his own theory of the unconscious.

In the current number of the *International Journal of Psycho-Analysis*,† he discusses the subject of

* Quoted by Dr Mitchell, p. 177.
† 1 Vol. III., No. 3.

" Dreams and Telepathy."   Most of the " telepathetic "
messages recorded by Myers entered consciousness in
the dream state.   His explanation for this, as we saw,
was that during the day, when consciousness is active,
the message is prevented from emerging from the
subliminal and so remains latent until proper conditions
are present.   Freud in the paper referred to examines
some dreams purporting to be the result of telepathic
messages, and, without deciding whether or not
telepathy be true, shows how their contents can be
explained by the psycho-analytic conception of the
unconscious.   His main contention is that whether the
dream be interpreted telepathically or not it need make
no difference to our conception of the unconscious.   If
telepathy be not involved we have to assume that the
thoughts of the previous day become reinforced by an
unconscious wish.   If telepathy is involved then the
" telepathic message has been treated as a portion of
the material that goes to the formation of a dream like
any other external or internal stimulus " (p. 292).
This is very important, for whether or not telepathy can
be dispensed with, it suggests that we can dispense
with Myers' Subliminal II. for such a theory as Freud
himself propounds.   There would be little advantage in
this unless it brought nearer that co-ordination of
widely differing phenomena, which Myers aimed at but
failed to accomplish.   The most that can be said at the
moment is that the evidence is strongly in support of
this possibility.   It is significant that by far the greater
number of telepathic presentiments and spiritistic
messages relate to the death of relatives, and this
accords with the finding of psycho-analysis that often
very strong " death wishes " against dear relatives are
harboured in the unconscious.   A case in point is
discussed by Freud in the paper we have been referring
to.   He cites, amongst many telepathic experiences of
a correspondent, the following : " In 1914 my brother

47

was on active service ; I was not with my parents in B but in C. It was ten in the morning on August the 22nd when I heard my brother's voice calling ' mother, mother.' It came again ten minutes later, but I saw nothing. On August the 24th I came home, found my mother greatly oppressed, and in answer to my question she said, that the boy had appeared on August the 22nd. She had been in the garden in the morning, when she had heard him call ' mother, mother.' I tried to comfort her and said nothing about myself. Three weeks after there came a card from my brother, written on August 22nd between 9 and 10 in the morning ; shortly after that he died."

The following passage contains Freud's attempt to relate this experience to his psycho-analytic principles : " It cannot be proved but also cannot be disproved that instead of this what happened was the following : the mother told her one day that her son had sent this telepathic message ; whereupon the conviction at once arose in her mind that she had had the same experience at the same time. Such delusory memories arise in the mind with the force of an obsession—a force derived from real sources—they have, however, substituted material for psychical reality. The strength of the delusory memory lies in its being an excellent way of expressing the sister's tendency to identify herself with the mother. ' You are anxious about the boy, but I am really his mother, and his cry was meant for me ; I had this telepathic message.' The sister would naturally firmly decline to consider our attempt at explanation and would hold to her belief in the authenticity of the experience. She simply cannot do otherwise ; as long as the reality of the unconscious basis of it in her own mind is concealed from her she is obliged to believe in the reality of her pathoganic logic. Every such delusion derives its strength and its unassailable character from its source in unconscious psychical reality."

48

This explanation leaves the experience of the mother untouched, and telepathy may or may not have operated in her case. Freud's only concern is to show that in the case of the daughter, who reported her experience to him, the unconscious, as he conceives it, might well be its source.

The real value of an attempt to apply the principles of psycho-analysis to " psychical " phenomena is that when the work is thoroughly done the spiritistic and telepathic hypotheses can no longer hang in the air. Either they will be accepted as sound and necessary principles or else they will be completely discredited.

Our reason for this statement is that psycho-analysis has placed in the hands of the investigator methods of exploring the unconscious that until recently were unknown. With the aid of these principles all the contents of the unconscious can be raised to consciousness. In this way it can be discovered whether the so-called supernormally acquired knowledge has or has not its source in the unconscious. The crucial test would be to analyse the medium or the subject of " telepathic " communication. If this were done in the Doris Fitscher case or in the case of those whose experiences Freud reports, the results might or might not be different, but they would be offered with much greater conviction. There is obviously one great difficulty to be surmounted in the actual work of analysis. The psycho-analysis of any person cannot be carried out without that person's honest co-operation, and it cannot be hoped that this will be easy of attainment in every case. Since, for example, the medium in the course of analysis may lose her " gift " through a synthesis of the sundered elements of the personality, it is not likely that co-operation with the analyst will be possible. But if this difficulty can be avoided, then the position either for or against spiritualism and telepathy will be fairly well established.

CHAPTER III

THEORIES of the type now to be considered differ fundamentally from those described in the previous chapters, having been developed from the study of hysteria in its various forms. So also have those theories which are associated with psycho-analysis. We are, however, in this chapter to confine our thoughts to the views of those who treat mental disorder, and seek to effect healing, by a different method from that adopted by psycho-analysts.

The chapter will consist of three sections. The first will be devoted to matters of a more or less general kind. It will refer to the importance of the discovery that hysteria is often functional, and not organic, in its ætiology, and that, therefore, psychological, not physiological, methods of healing are correct. The second section will take into account the nature of the evidence for the *existence* of the subconscious, which a study of the phenomena of hysteria affords. In this connection the evidence (i) from the phenomena of certain automatisms, (ii) from those of multiple personality, (iii) from those of suggestion, will be noted. This section will be followed by another in which brief accounts will be given of the *theories* of the subconscious held by Pierre Janet, Boris Sidis, and Morton Prince.

I

Janet in many of his works emphasises the importance of the discovery that the ætiology of some forms of mental trouble is purely psychological. Owing to a misunderstanding with regard to this, on the part of earlier physicians, patients experienced needless suffering. Many of them had limbs removed in a vain effort to produce health, others underwent prolonged treatment, which, in the end, brought no relief, while many were compelled to spend their days in an asylum, who, with a different method of treatment, might have become useful members of society.

The discovery that many forms of hysteria are wholly psychological took place in connection with the researches of a group of physicians into cerebral localisation. These researches led to such interesting and valuable results that, as Jung says, " everyone began to go in for post-mortem examination." Amongst other results these examinations revealed the fact that out of a number of patients examined in an asylum more than half were not suffering from brain defect, and yet were insane. From this it was concluded that the real factors in the causation of a large proportion of mental troubles were not physiological at all, but psychological.

Certain French writers, especially Liebault and Bernheim of the first Nancy School, Charcot and Pierre Janet, established beyond all doubt the truth of this by the aid of many ingenious experiments. It was found, for example, that in the case of hysterical paralysis of the legs, if a patient could be induced to forget his trouble, he was able to walk and even run. Baudouin, of the New Nancy School—to the principles of which attention will be given in the next section—records the case of a woman, who, for many years, was a sufferer from paralysis of the legs and was bed-ridden. On one occasion her house went on fire, and in the highly emotional situation that followed, she jumped out of bed and ran downstairs. Asked afterwards to explain how she got herself into safety, she declared that she did not know. Cases of this kind prove that there is nothing wrong with the legs—the trouble is not organic but psychological. In another respect this is clear. A patient who suffers in this way will declare, for example, that his leg is completely paralysed, or is paralysed up to the knee. But when the affected part is compared with the rest of the leg there is no anatomical difference. The part supposed to be paralysed is not shrunk or withered, as it would be if real organic paralysis had set in. So far as the patient's power goes the leg is paralysed, but not in the ordinary way through the spine. Both the paralysis itself and the area paralysed correspond to the subject's own crude notions. The only reasonable conclusion is that it is the *idea* of the leg that is the determining factor in these cases.

This discovery led, of course, to a revolution in the methods of treating hysterics. It is in connection with the study of these new methods that light has been thrown upon the existence and nature of the subconscious.

II

Let us first consider the evidence for the *existence* of the subconscious. The whole field of evidence, of course, cannot be surveyed here. We shall confine our attention to three types of phenomena-motor automatisms, multiple personality and suggestion.

(i) The evidence from *Motor Automatisms*—

Experiments carried out by Janet and others on patients suffering from hysterical anæsthesia yield us interesting illustrations of this phenomenon. Let us give a short account of his experiments on anæsthetic arms.

Patients suffering in this way do not consciously feel pain in the affected arm. They declare the arm to be quite insensible. Any stimulus, such as the pricking of a pin, may be freely applied, but so long as the eye of the patient is on the arm no reaction takes place. If, however, the arm be hidden from the patient and the stimulus then applied reaction takes place, showing that the arm is not really devoid of feeling, but that, on the other hand, the patient feels subconsciously. Janet experimented in this way with the help of a screen that kept the hand hidden from the patient, and it was found that the subject evinced not only susceptibility to pain, but also to suggestion. Thus, when the hand was gently moved backward and forward it continued to move by itself. When raised it tended to remain in an upright position for a time. When a pen was placed between the thumb and the forefinger, the hand generally closed upon it in the way adapted for writing. When the fingers were guided to write certain letters, and the hand of the experimenter was then withdrawn, the patient often continued to write until a whole sentence was produced. When a word was misspelled the patient's hand frequently hesitated, and sometimes rewrote the word correctly.

The point contended for in experiments of this kind is that since apparently *purposive* movements take place of which the primary consciousness is unaware, another consciousness, or quasi-consciousness, must control the various movements of the subject. Without such an hypothesis the behaviour of the hysteric would be unaccountable.

Janet has gone further: he has claimed that he has been able to get into direct communication with this " secondary consciousness." He has adopted the method of " distraction." Even in normal cases, if the mind is strained in its attention to any object or occupation, it becomes oblivious to physical surroundings, and can be induced in this condition to produce complicated movements, without conscious awareness. But the extent to which this is done in normal persons is limited, as compared with the extent to which it is possible in the hysterical subject. Janet has found that in the latter case while one engages the patient in conversation, another may quietly come behind him, and, by whispering suggestions into his ear, get him to perform various movements, and even answer questions by writing or gesture.

We shall leave this sort of argument for the unconscious with the remark that some of the movements recorded may very well be explained as habitual or automatic. " Behaviourist " psychologists are teaching us that very complicated types of activity can be explained, even without the concept of consciousness, as due to habit—habit being considered as a physiological process. But when one reads the accounts of these experiments fully and considers what they seem to reveal, one finds it difficult to explain the phenomena without some theory of the subconscious. There are other phenomena, the nature of which we shall now indicate, that go to confirm this view.

(ii) The evidence from " Multiple Personality "—

The phenomenon of multiple personality is of very great importance from the standpoint of the subconscious. A number of important cases have recently been studied by physicians and psychologists. These reveal such definite alterations in temperament and character from time to time as to suggest that the " normal " personality is, for the time being, replaced by an entirely different one.

In the preceding chapter an account was given of the Doris Fitscher case of multiple personality, but there are many others on record, by far the most famous of which is that described by Dr Prince in his *Dissociation of a Personality*—the case known as " Sally Beauchamp."

THEORIES OF THE SUBCONSCIOUS

According to Dr Prince, Miss Beauchamp revealed no extraordinary abnormalities up to late adolescence, but she showed signs of an extremely nervous disposition, and was highly sensitive to every sort of impression. At the age of twenty-three, when she came under Dr Prince's care, she was an enthusiastic and successful student at college. She was, however, beginning to reveal signs of personal instability. This developed until the stage was reached when she could change her personality from day to day and, often, from hour to hour. With each change her character was different as were also her memories.

Altogether four personalities began to alternate with one another—the original and three others. All the personalities inhabited the same body, yet they were entirely different in character, in temperament, in thought, in habits, in memories, and in general culture. They seemed to differ in every respect as widely from one another as do distinct individuals that inhabit each a different body. Two of these personalities have no knowledge of each other or of the third, except such knowledge as they receive second-hand or by inference, and the memories of any two seem to be a complete blank while the other is in control. When one personality makes its appearance its life is not continuous with those it has replaced—but with its own previous life. It has to take up life from the point it has reached when it withdraws and the others come into existence. One of the personalities, known as Sally, differs from the others in that she has knowledge of them; she is represented, for example, as manifesting a strong dislike to the original personality—the real Miss Beauchamp. Her only concern seems to have been to cause the latter all the discomfort that is possible. Miss Beauchamp had an abhorrence of insects and reptiles; Sally during her absence provided her with a box, which when opened was found to contain six spiders. Sally herself was present "subconsciously" to witness the joke and states that when Miss Beauchamp opened the box she screamed, and the spiders ran all over the room. Miss Beauchamp did not like long walks, and became easily fatigued, but when Sally was in evidence she would take long walks into the country, and then disappear, leaving Miss Beauchamp to wake up and find her way back. Often Sally sought to do bodily violence to Miss Beauchamp ; but yet there seem to have been occasions when she repented of all this, and she left behind for Miss Beauchamp messages of friendliness.

The differences between Sally and Miss Beauchamp were enormous. The former lacked culture, the latter was highly cultured. Sally had knowledge of Miss Beauchamp's habits of life, but not of her mental equipment or attainments.

We have confined our account of the case to two personalities, but there were two others as well. The first of these was discovered when Miss Beauchamp was hypnotised ; the second came suddenly into the ascendancy after Miss Beauchamp had been about five years under Dr Prince's care. The point to be emphasised is his own account of the distinctive characteristics of each personality. "Each has a distinctly different character ; a difference manifested by different trains of thought, by different views, beliefs, ideals, and temperaments and by different acquisitions, tastes, habits, experiences, and memories."

Another case of a different type may be briefly summarised. It differs from the Beauchamp case in many respects. Instead of four personalities alternating with one another, there are only two. Instead of frequent alternations between these, only one is recorded to have taken place, and between the two personalities there is no communication of any kind.

The case is that of Rev. Ansel Bourne recorded by

William James. This man drew 551 dollars from a bank
in Providence, got into a car, and, immediately, lost
his sense of personal identity. He did not return home
that day, and was soon announced in the papers as
missing. The police engaged in a careful search for
him, but the search was fruitless. After two months
a man at Norristown, Pa., who had been calling himself H. J. Brown, and who had rented a small shop,
stocked it with stationery, confectionery, fruit, and
small articles, and had for two months carried on a
successful business, woke up suddenly, in a fright, and
called together the people of the place to know where he
was and how he got there. He told them that his name
was Ansel Bourne, that he was entirely ignorant of
Norristown, that he knew nothing of shopkeeping, and
that the last thing he remembered was drawing money
from the bank in Providence. That two months had
elapsed since that occasion he could scarcely believe.
The people regarded him as insane, and his nephew
came to bring him back to his home.

Here we have the case of two very distinct
personalities—one completely replacing the other for
a time — revealing tendencies, desires, and aptitudes
that were entirely foreign to the other.

The end of the story of the Beauchamp family was
that by hypnotism all the personalities became united
into the original. But in the case of Ansel Bourne
this was not possible. William James found that in
hypnotism he could have the Bourne personality restored, but he did not succeed in having it merged into
the original personality. He finishes his story by saying: " I had hoped by suggestion to run the two personalities into one and make the memories continuous,
but no artifice would avail to accomplish this, and Mr
Bourne's skull to-day still covers two distinct personal
selves." *

* *The Principles of Psychology*, Vol. I., p. 392.

Now, for the elucidation of the phenomena of multiple personality modern psychology regards some theory of the subconscious as absolutely necessary. When one of these " personalities " has disappeared it has not ceased to exist but forms the subconscious. Sometimes, however, as in the case of Miss Beauchamp, there is a co-existence of two personalities.

I have chosen Miss Beauchamp and Ansel Bourne as examples of multiple personality because the one points to the existence of what Dr Prince calls " co-consciousness," while the other only points to what may be called " alternating consciousness." Sally was sometimes capable of recognising the dominant or conscious personality—the real Miss Beauchamp—and we have, therefore, the case of two " personalities " existing at the same time. In most cases, however, we have evidence only of the existence of one personality at a time—though the fact that it is replaced frequently by another shows that the other existed all the time in some form. The two types of multiple personality, however, lead to different interpretations of the subconscious.

The cases we have described are very exceptional. In the whole of modern psychological literature not more than a dozen such cases are recorded. Those which we have described—with the Hanna case of Dr Sidis—are the best known. It may, therefore, be objected that it is not legitimate to draw any inferences as to the subconscious from such a limited number of hysterical cases. The answer is that it is quite legitimate to draw conclusions as to the existence of the subconscious in the limited number of cases studied. In these particular cases a subconscious does manifest itself ; but it is quite just to argue that from these cases we have no right to draw conclusions as to the existence of the subconscious in normal cases. This point, however, is largely neutralised by the contention of modern psychologists, and physicians, viz., that we cannot draw a hard and fast line between the normal and the abnormal—these are but relative terms. According to this view, then, we must regard the cases of multiple personality which we have referred to as only extreme developments of what is characteristic of all "normal" individuals. In other words, the minds of the normal are not quite so unified as was at one time supposed. Dr Sidis has laboured this point at great length in his *Multiple Personality*.

The general truth of this contention must, I think, be conceded, but it must be stated with great caution. It must not suggest more than the fact that the same individual may experience at the same time opposing impulses or conflicting mental tendencies, and that in certain conditions the tendencies that we habitually repress may take control for a time, to be repressed again by the opposing tendencies. We shall give some examples of this from experiences that are quite common. It should be noted that while these reveal in the self antagonistic tendencies, they do not reveal deep dissociation accompanied by amnesia such as characterised the Beauchamp or Bourne case. A suitable example of what we mean is the state of intoxication and what it reveals. There is often such a difference of character and general behaviour between the two states—drunkenness and sobriety—of the same man, as to suggest an alternation of personality.

Again, in dreams we are often represented as different from what we are in waking life. Nearly everyone has at some time dreamt himself to be some one else ; and it may be argued that, for the time being, he was not himself—a temporary break up of his personality took place.

To some extent alterations of personality take place with great frequency in the normal waking state. We all have our moods. Our states of thought and feeling are by no means constant. With every change of mood there is a change in attitude towards others, manifesting itself in unaccountable good humour, or ill-temper. Human nature often reveals a wonderful capacity to change with great suddenness from one of these to another.

Perhaps, however, no phenomena are more important in this connection than those commonly called religious. We introduce them here because of their close relationship to multiple personality, and because of the inferences to be drawn from them with regard to the subconscious.

In a recent number of the *Hibbert Journal* * a writer describes his experiences when faced with death. Normally, he tells us, he had an unusual dread of death, and a great passion for life. But on one occasion, at the prospect of immediate death, he says: " For one instant terror possessed me, then amazement, at the nearness of death. I forgot fear, and was conscious of a faint but distinct sense of exultation. During those instants no . imagination of the pain of death, no thought of the meaning of death in itself came to me. Wonder and exultation like a sound heard from a great distance filled my mind. Life was simply ' what is,' death ' what is not.' Life was full of sane, healthy joy. But gladness, faint and indescribable, came with the nearness of death. . . . The fact that in a few minutes I might be drowned caused me no fear and no shrinking, rather a sense of well-being and faint triumph." This and many other similar experiences are described by the writer for the explanation of which he draws on the conception of a dual consciousness. " It was not my normal self that face to face with death felt only exultation, forgot fear, and desired most of all to spare my friends suspense and sorrow. Another self had dominated my conscious self during those instants. That self

* Vol. IX., No. 1.

saw death, personal pain, and separateness as illusion."

Probably, if the writer were less philosophical he would have referred such experiences to an external supernatural source as their explanation. As it is he sees in the experience a manifestation of a consciousness that cannot be identified with the primary consciousness of his previous life.

William James in his *Varieties of Religious Experience* gives the record of many whose personalities were completely altered, who, to use religious terminology, experienced " sudden conversion." Examination of these cases disclosed the fact that the state preceding conversion—especially sudden conversion—is one in which the individual is conscious of imperfection, and want of inward unity, as if there were two diverse sets of tendencies and emotions—one striving against the other. In St Augustine's *Confessions* we have a noteworthy example : " The new will which I began to have was not yet strong enough to overcome that other will strengthened by long indulgence. So these two wills, one old, one new ; one carnal, the other spiritual, contended with each other and disturbed my soul. I understood by my own experience what I had read, ' flesh lusteth against spirit and spirit against flesh.' It was myself indeed in both the wills, yet more myself in that which I approved in myself than in that which I disapproved in myself. Yet it was through myself that habit had attained so fierce a mastery over me, because I had willingly come whither I willed not. Still bound to earth, I refused, O God, to fight on Thy side, as much afraid to be freed from all bonds, as I ought to have feared being trammelled by them." *

In the phenomenon of multiple personality hypnotic suggestion is the means usually adopted to bring about

* *Confessions*, Book VIII., chap. v. Quoted by William James in *Varieties of Religious Experience*, p. 172.

unity and harmony. But in the case of the religious phenomenon of the " divided self " inward harmony and sense of completeness are brought about by " conversion." These methods, however, are not essentially different. The New Nancy School contends that conversion is a form of auto-suggestion—and hypnotic suggestion also must be reduced to auto-suggestion before it can be effective.

The main point, however, is that the phenomena we have been referring to point to the existence and activity of the subconscious. This is recognised, not only by modern psychologists who regard conversion experiences as forms of hysteria, but by theologians who will not admit this. Professor James' explanation of conversion—put in psychological terminology—is as follows : It is " due largely to the subconscious incubation and maturing of motives deposited by the experiences of life. When ripe the results hatch out or burst into flower." *

(iii) Evidence from the Phenomena of Suggestion—

Suggestion in various forms is the method adopted by a great number of medical psychologists for the cure of hysteria. It was the method adopted by the pioneers in psychological treatment such as Charcot, Liebault, and Bernheim. It is the method employed still by Pierre Janet and other French physicians. Leading American physicians such as Drs Boris Sidis and Morton Prince also make good use of this method. But it is to the New Nancy School, of which Coué and Baudouin are the leaders, that we must turn for the best account of the working and results of this psycho-therapeutic method. Let us, therefore, give an exposition of the principle of this school—at the same time bringing

* *Varieties of Religious Experience*, p. 230.

out the main points of difference between this latest form of the method of suggestion and those that preceded it. It will be seen that the phenomena of suggestion point to the existence and activity of the subconscious.

The first Nancy School, of which Liebault and Bernheim were the founders, recognised two distinct factors in all suggestion : (i) The presence of an operator who suggested ideas to the subject—the latter usually being first brought into the hypnotic state. (ii) The reception of the idea by the subject, and its transformation into the corresponding reality. It was the former of these factors that was regarded by the earlier experimenters as the essential in suggestion. The New Nancy School, however (i) regards the presence of the operator as non-essential ; (ii) regards hypnosis—especially deep hypnosis—as unnecessary ; (iii) accepts as of the essence of suggestion the transformation of the idea into reality, but adding, as of the greatest importance, that this takes place in the subconscious. Let us elaborate these three points.

(i) The presence of an operator is non-essential to suggestion.

This means that auto-suggestion becomes the type of all suggestion. Before hetero-suggestion can be successful it must be transformed into auto-suggestion, *i.e.*, it must be accepted by the subject and made his own. No hetero-suggestion is ever successful if it is opposed to the conscious tastes and desires of the subject. If the subject has conscious standards of goodness, any suggestion that is inconsistent with these will not be carried out. On the other hand, the reason why health suggestions from an experimenter are nearly always successful is that they are generally in harmony with the patient's desires. We say generally in harmony—because psycho-analysis is showing how frequently the patient does not really want to get better, though he would not admit this to himself. In such circumstances hetero-suggestion cannot be realised. It meets with a counter-suggestion in the patient's subconscious and this acts as an inhibiting barrier to the transformation of the idea. This has been borne out by experiments wrought even on subjects in the hypnotic state. Here one would imagine that the operator would be the chief factor and that no counter-suggestion could arise in the mind of the subject. But the following favourite experiment of Coué's indicates that the case is otherwise. " He suggests that the subject should see an apparition clothed in white on the right-handed window pane. As he makes this suggestion he thinks of the upper pane on the right side. The subject will see the apparition on one of the right-hand panes, but it will be, in most cases, on the lower pane—the one through which he usually looked out. If the suggester, though he has said the right-hand pane, has wrapped this up in a number of details so that the right-handedness may readily be overlooked, it is quite likely that the subject will see the apparition upon a left-hand pane. As for the aspect of the apparition each subject will describe this according to his own fancy. This proves beyond dispute that what is realised is not the thought of the hypnotiser. The subject has heard the latter's words and has interpreted them as would a person in the waking state. . . . He sees what he has thought—not what the hypnotiser has willed." *

The thesis upon which the New Nancy School in this way insists, viz., that auto-suggestion is the type of all suggestion, goes a long way towards meeting the objection brought against the earlier statements of the theory, viz., that it involved the enslavement of the subject to the will of the experimenter, the complete

* *Suggestion and Auto-Suggestion*—Baudouin, pp. 200-201.

suppression of one's own individuality. The new teaching, so far from involving anything so degrading to the personality, implies the very opposite. It advocates the method of auto-suggestion for the purpose of developing all mental faculties—memory, attention, will, etc. Thus, like the psycho-analytic method, the principles of the New Nancy School are regarded as not only applicable in the sphere of mental disease, but also in the domain of education, and as of great importance in every-day life.

Before passing away from this first, and most important principle of the New Nancy School, let us see what further light may be cast upon it by a brief reference to the mode of procedure adopted by physicians who practise this method. Every patient who presents himself for treatment in the hospital at Nancy is first taught the art of auto-suggestion. He is put through preliminary exercises in order that the power of suggestion may be demonstrated to him, and that he may be convinced of its value. The subject is told that his mind is like soil that has to undergo a course of treatment before the seed to be sown in it can germinate. When the patient is convinced of the effectiveness of this method he then receives further instructions as to how suggestion may be carried out. He is told to make general suggestions to himself rather than particular ones. Instead of a special suggestion being recommended for each slight or serious ailment, the patient is urged to suggest something like the following : " Day by day, and in every way, I am getting better and better." Positive suggestions rather than negative ones are recommended. Instead of suggesting to oneself that the disease is passing away it is better to suggest that the signs of growing health are fast appearing. Suggestions of the latter kind turn the mind to the goal of health and away from disease—a matter of great importance.

E

From these hints with regard to methods of procedure it will be obvious that the main aim of the New Nancy School is to render each patient capable of curing himself. In hetero-suggestion patients depend too much on the physician, and the cures wrought are not always permanent ; but by teaching the patient to adopt a certain mental attitude towards himself and towards life, and to practise regular auto-suggestion, permanent cures are more often effected. Coué tells us that he frequently addresses his patients on their first visit as follows : " You have come here in search of someone who can cure you. You are on the wrong track. I have never cured any one. I merely teach people to cure themselves. I have taught many to cure themselves, and that is what I am going to teach you." *

The first principle of the New Nancy School, therefore, is that auto- and not hetero-suggestion is the type of all suggestion.

(ii) In the second place, the New Nancy School regards the deep hypnosis, on which other experimenters in the same psycho-therapeutic method depended so much for results, as non-essential. Hypnosis is not abandoned altogether, but it is recommended, if at all, only in its lighter forms. Deep hypnosis had to be abandoned owing to its inconsistency with the principle that auto-suggestion is the type of all suggestion. For deep hypnosis is always characterised by amnesia in the waking state. When the patient wakes from the trance he has no memory of what took place during the sleep. For this reason the suggestions made during hypnosis could not be deliberately carried out, i.e., reflective auto-suggestion would be absent. What are the mental conditions that the New Nancy School proposes to substitute for that of " induced sleep " ? The one factor essential to successful auto-

* *Op. cit.*, p. 220.

suggestion is complete mental relaxation involving an absolute suspension of the will. This latter point is central in the teaching of the New Nancy School. " Never," says Coué, " let the will intervene in the practice of auto-suggestion." * The mental condition that most favours the realisation of a suggestion is one of effortlessness. The idea itself must reach a high degree of intensity. This, however, is not brought about by an effort of will, but by a contraction of the field of consciousness. An idea—when competing ideas are absent—holds the attention instead of the attention holding it.

Coué and his school place the will at a discount owing to the " law of reversed effort." By this is meant that conscious effort, if the imagination is adverse to it, or a counter-suggestion is at work, will only reinforce the counter-suggestion, and so will always end in a negative result. Everyone who has learnt to ride a bicycle, will be familiar with the truth of this. The inexperienced cyclist sees an object in his way. He tries to steer clear of it—but the greater his conscious effort to do so the more likely he is to fail. Similarly in, say, the case of health, when a cure is not brought about by suggestion, the probability is that a counter-suggestion—in the form of a fear of failure—is present. So long as this fear, which in itself is a spontaneous auto-suggestion, remains, a cure is impossible. Every conscious effort to get better only reinforces the counter-suggestion and the last state of the patient is worse than the first.

The patient, therefore, who wishes to adopt the method of auto-suggestion must train himself to an ignoring or suppressing of the will and to an exercising of the imagination, that is, to adopt a sort of free, effortless mental attitude—a relaxation not by changing the object of attention, but by a complete suspension

* *Op. cit.*, p. 125.

of attention. The patient is told that this condition is best favoured if he lies on his back, relaxes his muscles, and closes his eyes to prevent all distraction.

The condition just indicated as the most favourable to auto-suggestion is almost identical with that of reverie, which psycho-analysts consider of great importance. In this condition the mind is occupied with free ideas, and passes from one to another in quite an effortless way. The importance of mental relaxation is that it favours the entrance of subconscious material into consciousness. On this point the teaching of the New Nancy School is in agreement with that of psycho-analysis, and the influence of Bergson, who has worked out this point with great care, can be traced in both.

The foregoing points in the work of the New Nancy School only prepare the way for the third main point, which for our purpose is of the greatest importance.

(iii) The subconscious is an indispensable factor in explaining the phenomena of auto-suggestion. This fact is brought out in the definition of suggestion given by Baudouin. Suggestion is " an idea which undergoes transformation into an activity and the mechanism by which this is brought about is in the subconscious— suggestion is the subconscious realisation of an idea." *
According to this definition the sole function of consciousness in suggestion is to provide the idea or set the goal ; the subconscious finds the means to the fulfilment of the idea or of attaining the goal. Subconscious activity is, therefore, *teleological* in its nature. Upon this characteristic of the subconscious the New Nancy School lays great emphasis. " Suggestion acts by subconscious teleology. When the end has been suggested, the subconscious finds means for its realisation. In the search for experiments it often astonishes us by its skill and sagacity. All is grist which

* *Op. cit.*, pp. 25, 26.

comes to the mill and it has no scruple about cheating." *

The rôle of the subconscious in suggestion is illustrated by Coué and his school in a variety of ways. Thus in spontaneous auto-suggestion we are reminded of frequent experiences of difficulty in recalling a familiar name. The subject makes all sorts of efforts to recall the name—by trying to remember the number of letters in it, or the initial letters, etc.,—but without success. At length he turns his thoughts to other things and, later, when no attempt to recall the name is being made—" suddenly in the depths of our memory a call sounds resembling a telephone bell . . ., the connection we have been seeking is established, and the name is remembered." This is the result of subconscious activity which has been begun by the conscious effort to remember and continued when the subject was consciously engaged in other things.

Failures of memory of this kind the New Nancy School explains as due to the influence of some previous suggestion. This acts as a counter-suggestion and, in accordance with the law of reversed effort, every conscious attempt to have the name recalled produces only negative results. We shall see that psycho-analysis offers a different explanation when we come to deal with that subject.

Hartmann, we remember, illustrated the working of the unconscious by what may be called mental conversion. The New Nancy School makes use of the same phenomenon in support of subconscious activity. An opinion is presented to us. We either scornfully deny its truth or accept it with reserve. Time passes, and though in the meantime no further consideration has consciously been given to it, yet when again presented we find ourselves in complete agreement. What we had previously denied we now accept. The explanation is

* *Op. cit.*, p. 117.

that " the grain planted in him when he read has germinated in the subconscious." *

Similarly with the problems, which at night we leave unsolved and find easy of solution the next morning. The effort put forth during the waking state to solve the problem is transferred during sleep to the subconscious. Here the work goes on until the solution is found. Some psychologists refuse to admit that in this case there is any evidence of subconscious activity; the reason why our efforts meet with such ready success in the morning is that the mind is clear after rest. This explanation meets those straightforward cases where the problem is found on waking to be easily solved. But the school with which we are concerned presents us with complicated cases where the solution comes at midnight in the form of a dream, or where the patient awakes soon after falling asleep to find the problem solved. It is a fact, of course, that recuperation of the mind takes place very swiftly during the early part of sleep. But it is the waking up at an unusual hour, as though the subconscious arouses consciousness to communicate to it the news that the problem is solved, that has to be explained. It seems necessary in such cases to bring in the hypothesis of the subconscious.

Most people have experienced the fact that they can awake at any hour earlier than the usual one if only, on retiring, they make suitable auto - suggestions. Most people are also familiar with the fact that certain stimuli will arouse from sleep a person who may continue to sleep when intense stimuli of a different nature occur. The mother, for example, may sleep through the loudest thunderstorm, but is always aroused by the restlessness of her child. This seems to point in the direction of subconscious selective agency—responding to such stimuli as are connected with the welfare of the child.

One other phenomenon in this connection must be

* *Op. cit.*, p. 46.

mentioned—that of post-hypnotic suggestions. We do not get many illustrations of this in the literature of the New Nancy School for the reason already referred to : deep hypnosis is not advocated and seldom practised. Those, however, who still follow hypnosis as a psycho-therapeutic method provide us with many interesting illustrations from which inferences may be drawn to the existence of the subconscious. Dr Sidis, for example, relates how he suggested to a subject during hypnosis that on awaking, after a certain signal had been given, he should get up and walk round the room with an open umbrella in his hand The suggestion was carried out successfully. This is, perhaps, an extreme example. But it shows how even the most meaningless behaviour results from hypnotic suggestion. If the patient who is the subject of the suggestion is afterwards asked to account for his strange behaviour, he will seek as best he can to justify himself by rationalising, *i.e.*, by attempting a rational explanation which is not the real one, but which is the only one of which he is aware. The hypnotiser knows that the real explanation is that the subconscious takes control and carries out the idea presented to it in the trance. If we were dealing with only one of the foregoing considerations, it might be quite possible to dispense with the hypothesis of the subconscious ; but when taken together, and in conjunction with the wealth of phenomena brought to light by psycho-analysis, we have cumulative evidence for subconscious activity from which it is difficult to escape. We shall close this section by a reference to the fact that the teaching of the New Nancy School approximates—both in the importance of the rôle assigned to the subconscious, and of its activity—to the theories of the unconscious put forth by psycho-analysts.

In a recent address in this country * Coué has used

* Reported in the *Westminster Gazette*, 24th December 1921, from which this reference is taken.

the simile of a horse and cart to illustrate the relation of the subconscious to the rest of the individual. " Hitherto, our creaking wagon or our stately brougham has been drawn about in all manner of directions uncontrolled. Dr Coué has put the reins into our hands and experience will teach us how best to use them. Looking back we see that we have held the reins all the time, though we hardly knew how to use them. Now we can guide our cart." Leaving the simile aside, the New Nancy School, as well as the exponents of psycho-analysis, claims that with a proper control and use of the subconscious the manifold obstacles to happiness—unhealthy tendencies, bad habits, antipathies, passion, prejudice, hatred—can be all cleared away.

We shall now proceed to the third division of this chapter.

III

THE NATURE OF THE SUBCONSCIOUS

(i) The Theory of Janet—

The first important theory of the subconscious put forth in explanation of the phenomena of hysteria is that of Pierre Janet. It is generally conceded that this writer laid the foundations upon which later students of hysteria have built. We have already seen that to him in great part belongs the credit of discovering the fact that hysteria, in some of its forms, is psychologically explained. He was not satisfied, however, with this discovery, but went on to give a definite psychology of hysteria in which subconscious activity is involved. It is necessary at the outset to state that there is the greatest possible difference between the theory of the subconscious which we owe to Janet and all preceding theories. The early theories, we saw, were largely philosophical. But there is nothing of the speculative about the theory of Janet. He was a physician who attempted a purely scientific theory of the subconscious—a theory, that is, which was formulated out of a study of certain data, and which keeps close to the facts to be explained. In this respect it differs widely from the early theories. In this respect, also, it closely resembles the other theories to be considered in this and the next chapter. The influence of Janet's work may be clearly traced in these latter. They may go further and deeper than Janet's theory did, but the essential features of Janet's work can be traced in subsequent theories.

The term used by Janet is not the *unconscious* but the *subconscious*. Boris Sidis and Morton Prince make use of the same term, and it is, therefore, appropriate that we should treat all three writers together. The term is, on the whole, less objectionable than the term " unconscious " as employed by psycho-analysts. The latter term is often used in the sense of " unconscious consciousness," and when the objection is raised that this is a contradictory expression we are told that we must extend our conception of mind to include mental processes of which we are not conscious. The term subconscious as employed by Janet, Sidis, Morton Prince, and more recently by the New Nancy School, seems preferable, since these writers avoid such expression as " subconscious ideas." They speak of a subconscious self and subconscious personality, and these expressions, though objectionable, are not so obviously contradictory as that of " unconscious ideas."

There is an alternative expression very often used by Janet, viz., *secondary* consciousness. This expression is designed to meet the special phenomena of hysteria which he studies. The subconscious is more often applied by him to those mental states that form the margin of consciousness of the normal mind—the penumbra of consciousness as he calls it—than to the mental states of the hysteric. It is these latter states with which Janet was especially concerned, and to which he applies the term secondary consciousness. The phenomena of hysteria as he studied them require, he thinks, not only a subconscious in the sense of mental states existing outside the margin of consciousness, as they do in the case of the normal, but another consciousness analogous in every respect to the primary consciousness. This is his theory, and we have to ask how he accounts for it. By what processes does a secondary consciousness come into existence in the case of hysterics ?

It is clear, to begin with, that we do not bring a secondary consciousness with us into life. Only hysterics possess it, and hysterics as such are not born. Hysteria develops in the course of life. Those who turn out to be hystericals may bring predispositions in this direction with them into life ; but no one is actually born the subject of hysteria. No one, therefore, is born in the possession of a secondary consciousness such as we have evidence of in actual hysteria. Myers formulated a theory of the unconscious which, in one of its forms, we must assume is born with us and is an essential part of personality ; but the secondary consciousness of Janet's theory is not an essential part of personality. There is no evidence of its existence in the healthy minded. Some writers think that it can be discovered by hypnotism in the so-called normal, and they, therefore, argue that it can be found in all individuals, though it does not clearly manifest itself. It is not certain, however, that all individuals can become the subjects of hypnosis. Janet thinks that only hystericals can be hypnotised. If this be so our contention holds good—that secondary consciousness, as a form of the unconscious, is not to be found in the normally healthy. Moreover, if all men can be hypnotised it is quite possible that a secondary consciousness manifesting itself in the state of induced sleep may be brought about by suggestion, and, therefore, only exist during hypnosis.

If secondary consciousness develops only in connection with hysteria we have to ask how it is brought about. By what process is a secondary consciousness developed? This brings us to the main point in Janet's theory—*secondary consciousness is the result of dissociation.* In this process a part of consciousness gets split off from the primary stream of conscious life, becomes independent, and functions as a sort of separate personality, leaving the field of primary consciousness greatly narrowed. This process of dissociation is the common characteristic of all the symptoms of hysteria. In his book, *The Major Symptoms of Hysteria,* Janet brings this point out clearly. He goes through the list of symptoms, treating them one by one, and finds in them all the same characteristic—they all give evidence of a division of consciousness. Let us take the case of somnambulism, which is included in his list of the major symptoms. Somnambulism may be of two types: (i) monoideic. In this case one idea or group of ideas connected with one object gets split off from the main body of ideas and memories by which the primary consciousness is constituted. This split-off group of ideas takes on an independent life of its own, emancipating itself from the control of the waking conscious life. A case studied by Janet will serve as an illustration. Irene is the name of a girl who, in circumstances of extreme poverty, nursed her mother through a protracted and painful illness resulting in her death. Irene had not only to nurse her mother both by day and night, but she had the anxiety of having to meet all the financial needs of the home. This she attempted by working at intervals during the day. In these circumstances, with little sleep or nourishment, and with constant anxiety, her health became seriously undermined. Soon after her mother's death she fell into a nervous state in which she lived through again, on repeated occasions, the scenes and experiences of those trying days. She had complete amnesia as regards her mother's death, and thought she was still alive. She could hear her voice, and answer her questions, and relieve her wants as she did before the death took place. Interest in everything else completely vanished, and the girl was absolutely controlled by the one idea of attention to her dying mother. This one idea became split off from the rest of consciousness, the proof of this being that she did not remember her mother's death. One split-off partial system of ideas received an inordinate intensity and controlled her entire personality.

(ii) Janet distinguishes a different type of somnam-bulism to which he gives the name polyideic. This type of somnambulism differs from the foregoing in that it represents the splitting off from the main consciousness of more than one idea; also in this case emotional experiences may be dissociated. " In poly-ideic somnambulism it is a feeling in its entirety—a more or less precise feeling—that has separated from general consciousness and has developed in an independent way." * While many ideas may be involved in this type of somnambulism it would seem that they are all to be regarded as somehow interrelated by the one underlying feeling.

In polyideic somnambulism it often happens that the secondary consciousness gets adapted to its environ-ment, receiving impressions from the outside world, and reacting to them, as the primary consciousness does. This does not happen in monoideic somnambulism, in which the patient seems indifferent to external impres-

* The Major Symptoms of Hysteria, p. 65.

sions, except to those that may be directly related to the dominant idea. Fugues furnish us with illustrations of polyideic somnambulism in which the patient is capable of reacting to his surroundings in the same intelligent way as in the waking consciousness of normal life. A suitable case of fugue has already been described under the head, Multiple Personality, in this chapter. Ansel Bourne suddenly forgot who he was, assumed a new name, and for a fortnight wandered about from city to city. Then he settled down as a shopkeeper. Nothing unusual was noticed about him. He entirely forgot his former life. Then one morning he woke up and amnesia as regards the events of his secondary state took place.

It is not necessary to take the other symptoms of hysteria with which Janet deals to illustrate his theory. In some cases dissociation seems more definite than in others, but it is present as the common characteristic of them all ; in cases of functional anæsthesia dissociation only partially appears, e.g. it is clearer in tics and local paralysis, and it is very definite and complete in multiple personality.

In the cases we have given by way of illustration— those of Irene and Ansel Bourne—the chief thing to be noted is that the secondary consciousness has complete amnesia of the experiences associated with the primary consciousness. Likewise, when the primary state is resumed, amnesia for the experiences of the secondary state takes place, though these can be restored by hypnotic treatment. It is to this fact of amnesia that Janet especially appeals in proof of dissociation of consciousness. If the amnesia is reciprocal so that A is as ignorant of B as B is of A then the evidence of a split consciousness is clear enough.

So far the theory of Janet seems to be indisputable. The evidence seems unquestionably to point to the existence of what may be called a secondary consciousness. It is not necessary, however, for us to hold that while the secondary consciousness is in control the primary one exists, as such, subconsciously, or that when the primary state is restored the secondary consciousness continues to exist subconsciously. It is only necessary to hold that, while one state is dominant, the other exists subconsciously in the form of subconscious tendencies or dispositions. There are some cases, of course, that require a different explanation. These we shall notice when we deal with the theory of Dr Morton Prince.

When we ask the further question : How is dissociation of consciousness brought about ?, Janet's theory is not quite so satisfactory. Especially is this the case in the light of the work of Freud and his school. Janet's theory is that dissociation is due to a " lowering of the mental level." The consciousness of the normal healthy individual is capable of a high degree of synthesis and control. If I say " I feel a pain," " I see," " I feel that I move my arm," there takes place something that corresponds to the isolated words : " sensation of pain," " sensation of vision," " sensation of motion." But there is something more than these elementary phenomena in the statements, " I feel," etc. It is the " I " that makes the difference. Now this " I " consists of the union of all present sensations : " It is the notion of my body, of my capacities, of my name, of my social position, of the part I play in the world; it is an ensemble of moral, political, and religious thoughts. . . . There are, then, in the ' I feel ' two things in presence of each other—a small, new psychological fact . . . and an enormous mass of thoughts already constituted into a system—' I.' These two things mingle, and combine; and to say ' I feel ' is to say that the already enormous personality has seized upon and absorbed that little, new sensation which has just been produced. If we dared, . . . we should say that the ' I ' is

78

a living animal, extremely voracious, a sort of amœba, which sends out tentacles to seize and absorb a very small creature which has just been born at its side." *

Normally the individual is capable of discriminating between the various impressions that reach consciousness. He can, to a large extent, control and regulate his thoughts and desires. He has the power of reflection and will by which his conscious mental processes may be controlled. This capacity for control and " personal synthesis " depends on the maintenance of a certain level of nervous tension in the cerebral tissues. When this level falls too low the unity of consciousness is broken, and the personal synthesis becomes defective. " The subject has lost the mental synthesis that constitutes reflective will and belief ; he simply transforms into automatic wills and beliefs the tendencies which are momentarily the strongest. It is at that moment that the suggestions, the fixed ideas, the deliriums arise which complicate the disease during longer or shorter intervals." †

As factors in the lowering of the nervous tension by which the state of dissociation is brought about, Janet mentions the force of hereditary predispositions—and emotional shocks.

The weakness of this theory is that it gives us no explanation of the particular form that hysteria takes in any particular case. Supposing that there is a predisposition to hysteria, this does not explain why in one case the hysteria should take the form of a paralysed arm, in another case distressful vomiting or abstinence from food, and in another case loss of hearing or sight. Janet, for example, gives a long account of a case of hysterical blindness, but it is more descriptive than explanatory. Freudians get to the root of a case of this kind—or claim to do so—by explaining that

* *Op. cit.*, p. 305.
† *Op. cit.*, Introduction, p. 22.

the blindness is a self-imposed affliction in the nature of a penalty, for a perversion of one of the fundamental instincts. Whether the explanation in every case is correct or not it must be conceded that Freud's explanation of all forms of hysteria by the theory of repression is much more thorough than that of Janet. The latter falls back on hereditary predispositions and emotional shocks as the ultimate explanation of hysteria, the severance of consciousness being the result of these. The former admits the force of inherited predisposition in the production of hysteria, assigning to it, however, a subordinate rôle. The emotional shock he also admits as a factor in the case. But the all-important factor is the repressed emotional experiences of early life.

(ii) The Theory of Boris Sidis—

Dr Boris Sidis is one of the leading American exponents of the subconscious. He worked in the laboratory of Harvard at experiments mainly on hypnotised subjects. The nature and results of these experiments are set forth in his book *The Psychology of Suggestion*. He was also associated with Dr Goodhart in experiments on Multiple Personality, the results of which appear in a book of this title. It is to these two works we are indebted for the account of his theory which is given here.

Up to a point his theory seems to be identical with that of Janet, as the following quotation shows : " The law of suggestibility in general, and those of normal and abnormal suggestibility in particular, indicate a coexistence of two streams of consciousness, of two selves within the frame of the individual ; the one the waking consciousness, the waking self ; the other the subwaking consciousness, the sub-waking self." * The only difference between this statement of the subcon-

* *The Psychology of Suggestion*, p. 91.

scious and that of Janet is one of terminology. Janet speaks of a secondary consciousness. Sidis means the same thing, but the term he uses is the *sub-waking consciousness*—or the *sub-waking self*.

A large part of his work is taken up with the attempt to prove the existence of such a self. He denies that the theory of unconscious cerebration, as held by the older school of writers to which Carpenter belonged, can account for the facts. Memory itself is sufficient to discredit the adequacy of this theory. In memory the main factor is not the impression, conservation, or reproduction of experience, but its *recognition*. The theory of unconscious cerebration may account for the first three factors, but not for the fourth. In recognition an experience is not only reproduced but it is *recognised* as reproduced, *i.e.*, with the present experience there is a memory of a previous occasion when a similar experience took place. This Dr Sidis thinks unintelligible on a purely physiological account of the subconscious, for on such a view the trace of the earlier occurrence of the experience must be blotted out by the repetition.

A better proof of the existence of a sub-waking self offered by this writer is in certain experiments such as those referred to in the earlier part of the present chapter, viz., the movements of adaptation of the hysterical hand, etc. " It is obvious that in order that such movements of adaptation may occur there must be *recognition* of the object kept by the anæsthetic hand. But recognition requires a complex mental operation. It requires that the object should be perceived, should be remembered, and should be classed with objects of a certain kind and order." * It is not, however, with his proof of the existence of a sub-waking self that we are concerned but with its nature, and, as already stated, Dr Sidis seems to begin with a theory closely resembling that of Janet. *The difference between his*

* *Op. cit.*, p. 92.

theory and that of the latter writer—where difference exists—is rather one of application and development than one of kind.

(i) In the matter of *application* Janet did not assert the presence of a secondary stream of consciousness in the case of the normally healthy. His theory is applied to cases of hysteria only. Sidis, on the other hand, seems to hold that in all normal individuals there is a sub-waking self in addition to the waking self and that the difference between the normal and abnormal is that in the former there is a co-ordination of the two personalities, while this is absent in hysterical subjects. Two quotations will render his position clear. " The two selves in normal man are so co-ordinated that they blend into one. For all practical purposes a unity, the conscious individual is still a duality. The self-conscious personality, although apparently blended with the sub-waking self, is still not of the latter. The life of the waking self-consciousness flows within the larger life of the sub-waking self like a warm equatorial current within the cold bosom of the ocean. The swiftly coursing current and the deep ocean seem to form one body, but they really do not. The one is the bed in which the other circulates. The two do not mingle their waters ; and still they intercommunicate. The warmth of the Gulf Stream is conducted to the ocean, and the agitation of the ocean is transmitted to the Gulf Stream. So it is with the two selves." * " Multiple personality is not the exception but the law. . . . One great principle must be at the foundation of psychology and that is the synthesis of multiple consciousness in normal, and its disintegration in abnormal mental life." †

If we have to take the surface meaning of these

* *Op. cit.*, p. 162.
† *Multiple Personality*, p. 364.

quotations, viz., that in every normal individual there are, in addition to the waking self, one or more sub-waking selves, the latter being in nature analogous to the former, as the correct meaning, then we deny its truth. No one, I think, can reasonably deny that in the mind there are opposing tendencies, but this is very different from the view that in addition to the conscious self we are all in the possession of other selves of which for the most part we are unconscious. Dr Sidis does sometimes suggest a distinct difference between the waking and sub-waking selves. Thus the former possesses not only consciousness but self-consciousness. Also the term " sub-personal " suggests that the sub-waking self is less than personal. In *Multiple Personality* he explicitly states that the sub-waking self lacks a personality of its own, and that on this account it can readily assume the personalities of others. At one moment it is Luther, at another Mozart, Aristotle, or Plato.

These and other points of difference between the waking and sub-waking selves indicate that it is the statement of Sidis' theory rather than the theory itself that is at fault ; that all he means by a sub-waking self is the presence outside of consciousness of dispositions or tendencies that influence the conscious life and are influenced by it. It is this interpretation and this alone that we can accept as applicable in the sphere of the normal mind, and if it is a correct account of the position of Dr Sidis it would have been much clearer if different terminology had been employed. It is misleading and confusing to speak of a sub-waking self that lacks the characteristics commonly associated with a self.

(ii) There is a difference of *development* between the theory of Janet and that of Dr Sidis. The former simply distinguishes two separate streams of consciousness, or rather a division of the one conscious stream.

The latter goes further, defining more precisely the characteristics of consciousness as he conceives it, and of subconsciousness, and also distinguishing different levels or stages in the subconscious. The following are the outstanding points in his theory :

First, he conceives consciousness, and subconsciousness, as consisting in systems of " moments consciousness " arranged in a sort of hierarchy. Generally speaking a moment consciousness represents a single mental experience. He distinguishes a nuclear moment from other moments. The nuclear moment is the present, vivid experience that occupies the centre of consciousness. He speaks of it as the focus of consciousness and regards it as having a synthesising function. Like the amœba to which Janet compares consciousness the business of the nuclear moment is to gather to itself psychic material. Around this central moment " moments consciousness " arrange themselves in systems according to the degree of complexity which they possess. Thus there are groups, systems, communities, clusters, and constellations, each possessing a higher degree of complexity than the one preceding it. All these in the healthy mind are co-ordinated and synthesised, but it is possible for them to break up into their various moments, to become disaggregated. When this takes place we have what is known as mental " degeneration," such as is characteristic of hysteria, or is represented in the dream state. What happens in the former case is that under strong stimuli, such as traumatic experiences, dissociation of consciousness takes place, thus forming a secondary personality.

Dr Sidis emphasises the great influence of the subconscious moments not only in the mentally deranged, but in the mentally healthy. The moments that lie outside the focus " form the main sum of factors that determine indirectly the total psychic activity, they constitute the storehouse from which the central moment draws its material." *

The broad resemblance between the systems, etc., into which the moments consciousness are formed and the complexes of psycho-analysis is obvious. Psycho-analysts, however, limit the doctrine of complexes to the unconscious alone and also define more precisely than does Dr Sidis what a complex is. It is not merely a group of ideas, but a group of ideas emotionally toned and painful in nature. Dr Sidis' groups, clusters, etc., are simply arranged in order of complexity and we are not told of what mental element they consist or whether factors of all mental elements enter into their composition. On the whole, one infers that his systems of moments consciousness are entirely cognitive, and herein they differ from the complexes of the Freudian psychology.

One cannot avoid detecting in his theory the suggestion that the subconscious resembles in every way, except in degree of complexity, conscious states. The subconscious as well as the conscious consists of moments consciousness. Our contention is that there is a difference of kind between them—the subconscious consisting only of traces or tendencies left behind by experience.

The second main distinguishing factor in the theory of Dr Sidis is his division of the subconscious into the various states—hypnotic, hypnoid, hypnoidic, and hypnoidal.

Hypnotic states are such as are induced by hypnosis. They are highly suggestible. There is nothing that the hypnotic state will not accept when it is suggested by the experimenter. The hypnotic states reveal the subconscious as the slave of the hypnotiser.

This is not borne out, as we have seen, by the New Nancy School, in the teaching of which all suggestion

* *Multiple Personality*, p. 240.

is of the type of auto-suggestion. The hypnotised subject is not dominated by the experimenter, and only accepts from him those suggestions that fit in with the subject's general tastes and tendencies. Certainly many of the cases recorded by Dr Sidis help to bear this out. When the absurd is suggested it is only after repeated and authoritative commands that it is carried out.

Hypnoid states consist of the presence of two or more independent moments of consciousness. They are found in the phenomena of automatic writing and other kindred phenomena. In automatic writing, while the surface consciousness is otherwise engaged, as in conversation with someone, if a pencil is put into the hand of the subject he will write sentences and often whole paragraphs. The upper consciousness is entirely unaware of what is taking place, and there must, therefore, be a well-organised secondary consciousness controlling the automatic writing. Hypnoid states are " co-existing functioning dissociated states." *

Hypnoidic states are " outlived personalities." Whole phases of the patient's past life are lived over again. Unlike the hypnotic states hypnoidic states are not suggestible. The patient is preoccupied with his own past or with a phase of it ; he is shut off from his present environment. When a conversation, for example, is going on around him he takes no notice of it. These states are very unstable. As soon as the patient has lived through them they sink back into the subconscious. They are not induced artificially, but spontaneously break in on the flow of conscious life.

Hypnoidal states are outlived experiences—not outlived personalities. " The hypnoidal states are bits, mere fragments of past experiences." * They heave up from the subconscious with volcanic force and are neither recognised by the upper consciousness as part of

* *The Psychology of Suggestion*, p. 239.

past experience nor are they welcome. Unlike the hypnoidic states the hypnoidal states may be induced by the artificial process of " hypnoidisation." This method is practically identical with the Freudian method of " free association." The patient is asked to close his eyes and keep as quiet as possible, without, however, making any special effort to put himself in such a state. He is then asked to attend to some stimulus such as reading. When the reading is over the patient is asked, with his eyes still shut, to repeat it and tell what came into his mind during the reading or after it. In this way events, names of persons and of places, sentences, phrases, etc., wholly lapsed from memory, will often flash into the patient's mind. Hypnoidisation is a method of probing the patient's subconscious, and the result is always the release of bits of the patient's past experience. These form the hypnoidal states.

There are other states distinguished by Dr Sidis in the subconscious, such as the hypnoleptic. In this state the patient is unconscious and quiescent. He remains in an absolutely passive condition with his eyes firmly closed. But the most important of these states are the four we have mentioned.

I do not know that Dr Sidis has served any useful purpose in this effort to distinguish various states in the subconscious. The divisions he has made seem to be of an arbitrary nature, and, moreover, they lead him to adopt expressions that are confusing. In his effort, for example, to draw a clear distinction between hypnoidic and hypnoidal states he tells us that in the former " outlived personalities are resurrected " while in the latter one, bits of experience are restored to consciousness. The use of the word personality here for a phase of past experience—for this is all that it means on the theory of Dr Sidis—is very misleading. Unless terms are used with some degree of precision progress in the science of psychology is greatly hindered. Since the attention of psychologists has been directed to the study of hysteria the recognition of some division in the subconscious has been necessary ; but only one such division, it seems to me, is called for—that between the subconscious, which consists of traces of experience that can be voluntarily recalled to consciousness, and that which consists of traces, that can only be recalled by the help of a special method. In other words, the division which we owe to Freud seems to me necessary and at the same time sufficient.

IV

THE THEORY OF MORTON PRINCE

Dr Morton Prince is another American exponent of the unconscious, and his book, *The Unconscious*, is an important contribution to the subject.

The primary aim of this writer was to clarify the notion of the unconscious. In the theory of Sidis we found a lack of precision in the meaning of the terminology employed. The terms " sub-waking self " and " subconscious self " were scarcely appropriate when applied to mental processes that lack the chief characteristic of the primary conscious self. " Secondary self " can only be applied with any degree of appropriateness to certain manifestations of hysteria, and here another expression adopted by Dr Prince seems more appropriate.

Dr Prince justly points out the ambiguity in the use of the word " unconscious." Sometimes it is used for those mental processes of which we are unaware, while at other times it represents those processes that are entirely devoid of consciousness. These latter are again divided into unconscious mental processes and unconscious physiological processes.   Writers on the unconscious do not always make clear in which of these senses they use this term.   They are not always aware even that the term has any variety of meaning.   Dr Prince makes clear in what sense he employs the term. He limits its meaning to physiological processes, and applies a term of his own making to the mental processes and elements that are outside of ordinary consciousness. The term so employed is " the co-conscious."   *His theory, then, is a psycho-physiological one including both co-conscious and unconscious processes.   These two types of process are covered by a further term—the subconscious.*

(i) The Unconscious—

Dr Prince arrives at his definition of the unconscious as consisting in physiological factors by a careful analysis of the facts of memory.   Earlier writers, he thinks, have given but an inadequate account of all that memory involves.   They identify it with what is its last stage, viz., reproduction.   Memory, however, is not a product but a *process* in which there are at least three stages.   First, there is *registration*.   All experiences through which we pass leave impressions or traces behind.   This is true not only of the experiences of adult life, but also of those of childhood.   It is true not only of those events that occupy the centre of the field of consciousness, but also of those occurrences that have received but scant attention, and of which we were but dimly aware when they took place.   It is true not only of the experiences through which we pass in our normal mental states, but in the abnormal states as well.   Every impression received by the subject in the hypnotic trance is conserved and may influence him in unsuspected ways in his waking state.   All experiences of life leave behind their effects in some permanent way.

Secondly, there is the *conservation of experiences.*

89

The traces just referred to do not wear off ; they remain through the years and it is possible by the help of technical methods and devices, such as hypnotism, to have the experiences of early days recovered.

There is, thirdly, *the process of reproduction*—the recovery to consciousness of the registered and conserved experiences. Some identify this with memory, but, properly regarded, it is only memory's final stage.

Clearly, in the absence of any one of these factors there can be no memory ; there can be no conservation without registration, and both registration and conservation, whether for a shorter or longer period, are essential to reproduction.

Dr Prince adds that for " perfect memory " recollection is needed, by which is meant that we must recognise (re-cognize—cognize again) an event or experience as having taken place before. But we can have memory, he thinks, without this, and he cites in support of his view the results of many experiments in which experiences so entirely forgotten that they could never be *re*-cognised by the subject have been brought to consciousness. There has been recovery, but not recollection. Indeed, much of what we have experienced and is, therefore, conserved has never been actually attended to at all—it has only occupied the margin of consciousness, and hence cannot be recognised when reproduced.

We saw that Dr Sidis regarded recognition as the chief factor in memory and this seems to be the view commonly held. At the same time, the fact that experiences may be restored to consciousness without the possibility of recognising them as having taken place in the past is borne out, not only by the arguments of Dr Prince, but by the method of psycho-analysis. For the experiences that most influence us, according to the teaching of Freud, are those that occurred far back in childhood and so cannot be recognised, though their reproduction brings relief.

THEORIES OF THE SUBCONSCIOUS

Our author's limitation of the meaning of memory to this threefold process has enabled him to expound a purely physiological theory of the unconscious. His great objection to the theory of Dr Sidis is that it involves the conservation in concrete form in the subconscious of every idea, thought, and mental event that takes place in the course of life. Such a view he regards as absurd. Experiences are not conserved in the form in which they are present in consciousness. They are conserved only as traces or records in the neurones of the brain. Every experience modifies the neural arrangements and leaves behind neural records, so that if later any part of that particular neural system is stimulated the whole mental experience by which the particular arrangement was formed will be reproduced. To these systems, or traces, left behind as the result of experiences and capable of reproducing similar experiences when stimulated, Dr Prince gives the name " neurograms." Each neurogram is a storehouse of potential energy. When suitable conditions are present the potential becomes converted into the actual. The energy with which neurograms are charged is drawn from the innate tendencies and instincts around which they arrange themselves in systems. In this way subconscious processes of a highly complicated kind are brought about.

(ii) The Co-conscious—

If Dr Prince had confined his theory to the unconscious, as he had defined it, there would be little differences between it and unconscious cerebration ; but the work of Janet and Sidis, as well as other writers, rendered it necessary to introduce another concept for the explanation of phenomena for which the unconscious as a physiological concept could not account. For this purpose a highly appropriate term, the co-conscious, was adopted by Dr Prince. There are two sets of facts that this term is meant to cover.

First, it represents those ideas that exist at any time in the margin of consciousness of which we are but dimly aware. Everyone knows by introspection that there is a margin as well as a centre of consciousness and that the one shades off gradually into the other. Just as the centre shades off into the margin, so the margin, Dr Prince thinks, shades off into the ultra-marginal, and he assumes that in the ultra-marginal region as well as in the margin ideas exist as they do in the centre of consciousness. In the dim light of dusk objects that are close at hand may be seen in clear outline ; those further away more dimly ; while objects beyond a certain distance cannot be seen at all. These last exist all the same and have the same sort of existence as those that are visible. Similarly Dr Prince argues to the existence of ideas that are outside the margin of consciousness—ideas that possess the same sort of existence as those of which consciousness is clearly aware.

⸜ Dr Prince supports this view by an appeal to the results of hypnotic experiments. When by hypnosis the surface consciousness is removed, ideas in the subconscious break through. In post-hypnotic suggestion another proof is to be found, for here the subject carries out the idea suggested, though he is not conscious of the idea itself.

The present writer cannot help thinking that, in insisting on the existence of co-conscious ideas in the sense explained, Dr Prince is admitting what he has already denied. He objects to other theories of the subconscious because they involve the existence in concrete form of ideas once present in consciousness ; and this is unthinkable. Yet what is the co-conscious but the existence of ideas outside of consciousness in their concrete form ? Personally I do not think that any such ideas exist. It is doubtful whether ideas as such exist in the margin of consciousness for the marginal elements seem to undergo a change of some kind when brought into the centre. Attention makes some difference. This difference must either be one of degree or of kind. Either the marginal elements of consciousness are ideas dimly lighted up by consciousness or they are not ideas at all. The latter view seems to me the more likely. What exist in the margin of consciousness are psychical tendencies, and these become ideas when brought into the focus of attention. What is true of the margin is true also of the extra-marginal regions of the mind. In the first meaning attached to the term co-conscious, then, what exist outside of consciousness are not ideas, but psychical tendencies. Hypnotic experiments prove nothing to the contrary.

The second meaning of the term co-conscious is that of a " secondary consciousness " in the sense in which this term was used by Janet and Dr Sidis. We need not linger here except to say that we admit the presence of something like a secondary consciousness in some cases of hysteria. Already we have suggested that it is not necessary in cases of " alternating consciousness " —where one consciousness is followed by another, when both do not co-exist at the same time—to hold that while one consciousness is dominant the other must exist, as such, subconsciously. It is only necessary that it should exist in the form of tendencies ; these may become so strong, or the primary consciousness may become so enfeebled under shock or strain, that they break forth into a secondary consciousness, displacing the primary one.

This explanation, however, will not do where both streams of consciousness co-exist. It will not meet, for example, the Beauchamp case studied by Dr Prince. Sally was present subconsciously, while the real Miss Beauchamp was in control, not merely as a system of psychical tendencies, but as a self having a knowledge of the existence of Miss Beauchamp and making matters

93

as unpleasant for her as possible. I cannot see how, in this and similar cases, we can avoid the conclusion that something co-exists with the normal self, which represents a secondary consciousness. The application to this phenomenon of the term co-consciousness is exceedingly appropriate.

(iii) The Subconscious—

Dr Prince thinks it helpful to introduce another term by which the physiological and psychical processes that form his theory may be synthesised. For this purpose he makes use of the term subconscious. This term has been used by Janet and Dr Sidis in a psychological sense only. These writers, of course, do not ignore the physiological in their theories, but they treat physiological processes as do most psychologists, simply as correlates of consciousness, and not as parts of the unconscious to which their theories have reference. This seems to me on the whole a much sounder procedure than the one adopted by Dr Prince. It is well to keep the physiological and the psychological as much apart as possible. By so doing much better progress is likely to take place in both branches of science. Dr Prince, of course, is a neurologist and it is only to be expected that he should make the greatest possible use of physiological concepts.

SUMMARY

The main facts dealt with in the preceding pages of this chapter may be summed up in a few sentences. We have found in certain phenomena connected with the study of hysteria—motor automatisms, multiple personality, and suggestion—evidence for the existence of mental activity of which the primary consciousness is unaware. We have also considered the nature of this activity according to the theories of Janet, Sidis, and Morton Prince. The theories advanced by these

94

writers we call " subconscious theories," to distinguish them from the " unconscious theories " that underlie psycho-analysis. Some writers suggest that the main difference between these two types of theory is that the former type is based on the principle of dissociation and the latter on that of repression.* This is scarcely accurate since repression involves dissociation. The main difference in my opinion is the explanation given by each school as to why dissociation takes place.

Our main criticism of the theories considered is that the terminology used is misleading and unnecessary. Such expressions as " subconscious self," " subconscious personality," etc., are obviously objectionable, unless we are prepared to find more than one complete and independent personality inhabiting the same body. This is apparently not necessary when one is dealing with the normal mind. Subconscious dispositions as determinants of conscious activity are quite sufficient. We admit, however, that in certain cases of hysteria, especially in the Beauchamp type of multiple personality, something like a secondary consciousness is at work. It only remains to state that this admission does not necessarily involve a belief in the existence in these cases of two separate minds. There is but one mind. Primary and secondary consciousness are only expressions for distinct aspects of the mind that in very exceptional cases function separately and independently. That there was a unity in which the various " selves " of the Beauchamp family were different is proved by the fact that in the end they all merged into one, and the true Miss Beauchamp was rediscovered.

We have kept the consideration of Dr Prince's theory to the last because it seems to serve a suitable bridge to the next chapter in which we shall deal with psycho-analysis and the underlying theories of the unconscious. Janet and Sidis use the term subconscious alone ;

* Cf. *Psycho-Analysis*—Hingley, p. 15.

psycho-analysts make use only of the term unconscious. Dr Prince finds a place in his theory for both terms. Of course, as we shall see, there is little in common between his theory of the unconscious and those connected with psycho-analysis, but his general psycho-therapeutic method, if we were able to go fully into it, would reveal many points of affinity with the method of Freud. He, of course, practised hypnosis to discover the source of the symptoms of his patients ; but he did not depend solely on hypnotic suggestion to get rid of them. For this purpose he adopted the method of " re-education," which consisted of explaining to the patient the nature and meaning of his trouble, and advising him as to new attitudes to life. The general resemblance between this method and that of psycho-analysis is quite apparent.

CHAPTER IV

CONSIDERABLE rivalry continues to exist between the adherents of the " subconscious theories " considered in the preceding chapter, and the exponents of the " unconscious theories " to the consideration of which this chapter is to be devoted. Only a few years ago Janet published an article in the *Journal of Abnormal Psychology*, Vol. IX, in which he claimed that every principle in psycho-analysis had already found a place in his own theory, and that the difference between his theory and that of Freud was little more than verbal. Dr Ernest Jones, who is the leading exponent of the Freudian psychology in this country, replied that " the development of psycho-analysis both originated and proceeded quite independently of Janet's work, it was entirely uninfluenced by it throughout its whole course and would not have been different in one iota if Professor Janet's work had never existed." * These claims may be considered as extreme ; for there can be no doubt that Freud was well acquainted with the work of Janet. He, himself, acknowledges that he owes much to the work of Charcot and Bernheim, and Janet's theory is but a development of the former's. Just before Freud originated his great system he paid a visit to Paris, where the work of Janet was well known. It is unthinkable that he should not have been influenced by it. At any rate there is no great system

* *Papers on Psycho-Analysis*, p. 32.

that has not its roots in earlier work, and the theories we have been considering in the preceding chapter represent the soil in which psycho-analysis had its roots.

At the same time the originality and uniqueness of Freud's system must in all fairness be conceded. It differs quite definitely, for example, from the theories just considered in its abandonment of hypnosis and hypnotic suggestion as therapeutic agencies. For one thing, Freud found that not every patient suffering from functional diseases could be hypnotised, and, for another thing, treatment by hypnosis, when that was possible, only produced temporary relief. It may be quite a successful method of healing if the disease has been due to suggestion; otherwise the cures wrought in this way are superficial and the trouble quickly returns. Freud claims that his method has succeeded in cases where hypnotic suggestion had proved a failure. The reason for this will become obvious when we consider how complex the root of mental disorder often is. One of the great merits of psycho-analysis is that without the use of hypnosis it can go far down to the depths of the mind—which for psycho-analysts means going far back in the life of the individual—and discover in this way the root of the particular trouble.

Psycho-analytic, or " unconscious " theories, as they may be conveniently called, are based on the study of hysteria, as were the theories of the subconscious. It is necessary, therefore, that we should give some account of psycho-analysis before describing more in detail the types of unconscious theory on which it is based. Accordingly, our procedure in this chapter will follow that adopted in the preceding one. The first part of the chapter will deal with the evidence which psycho-analysis offers as to the *existence* of the unconscious. The second part will deal with the *types* of unconscious theory involved.

THE UNCONSCIOUS AND PSYCHO-ANALYSIS

I

The psycho-analytic method is the name given to the special means by which the memory is aided to reach the forgotten experiences of life, with a view to recalling to clear consciousness the details of emotional conflicts, which, although forgotten, exert an influence, often of an unfavourable sort, on the fortunes of one's life. Let us give an account (i) of the origin and development of this theory ; (ii) of the method employed for reaching the unconscious ; and (iii) of the differences that exist between Freud's theory and those theories that diverge from it.

(i) Origin and development of Psycho-analysis—

The first impulse to the development of psycho-analysis came from Dr Breuer of Vienna. He had occasion in 1881 to treat an intelligent patient suffering from an acute form of hysteria. With him was associated, as student and assistant, the one who was destined to become the founder of the new movement, Sigmund Freud. These investigators found that the facts offered by this patient in explanation of her trouble constituted only a small part of the story which in the end her memory succeeded in drawing from its depths. Each symptom of her trouble disappeared when the reminiscence connected with it was restored to memory. Thus she had lost the power to drink, and in the course of treatment an experience was recalled which took place immediately before this symptom first appeared. In the home of a governess whom she disliked she saw a little dog drink water out of a glass. This disgusted her very much at the time, but she said nothing about it and soon it was forgotten. Though forgotten it did not cease to exist ; it remained—or rather the emotion connected with it remained—in a " repressed " state in the unconscious. It was this repressed emotion that was the root of the particular symptom referred to.

When the memory of the occurrence was recalled, and she had re-lived it in its emotional intensity, the symptom disappeared. So it was with all the other symptoms. As the barrier was removed that had hidden the patient's past life from her present consciousness, and one forgotten emotional episode after another was recalled to her memory, her distressing symptom passed away.

Little was made of the experience gained from this case for a period of ten years, but Freud had been tremendously impressed by it, and, returning to Vienna after his period of training in France under Charcot, he persuaded Breuer to resume with him the investigation of other cases on the basis of the results obtained in this one. They continued to work together for a time. Then Breuer, seeing, as Freud says, that the researches were driving him in a direction in which he did not wish to go further, abandoned the work, and Freud continued the investigations himself. The result was the production of a theory that claims to be quite as revolutionary as the Darwinian theory of evolution, though in a different realm. Its importance is not confined to the clearer insight it gives into the nature of nervous troubles and how they may be cured. From the field of abnormal psychology it has extended its influence to general psychology, anthropology, folk-lore, religion, economics, criminology, sociology, history, politics, and biography. In all these departments of thought the working of unconscious motives is easily manifest to the trained psycho-analyst.

At first Freud was inclined to regard the traumatic experience as the chief factor in the ætiology of mental disorders. Soon, however, he came to the conclusion that this was not the only, nor the most important, factor to be reckoned with. Reaction to the shock, whatever its nature may be, depends on the person's temperament, hereditary tendencies, earlier mental history, and other conditions. The shock itself is not so much the cause as the occasion of the trouble, the real root of which usually lies in the forgotten experiences of childhood. These early experiences remain in the unconscious and add their emotional strength to the present painful experience. It is this that renders the traumatic occurrence important in the causation of the neurosis.

Having discovered in this way the importance of the early experiences of life Freud gave himself to a thorough investigation of the nature of child life. Upon the results of this study he has built up his whole system. He has discovered—and this is fundamental in his theory—that the unconscious in which is to be found the source of neurotic illness has been built up from infancy by the repression of experiences and impulses that, to the later developing consciousness, are seen to be painful. It is not the impulses in themselves that are painful; on the contrary, during the first years of life they are the only source of pleasure available to the child. But what society regards as natural in the child it will refuse to tolerate in the adult. Accordingly, as the child develops, the sources from which he derived gratification change to sources of pain. His methods of deriving pleasure become incompatible with the social and moral standards of civilisation and have, on that account, to be repressed. This repression goes on from the early years of life. Once the dawn of consciousness begins, the child is met with prohibitions from parents and others, so that its natural cravings and instincts are not allowed free expression. Early in life, therefore, the individual learns to control his impulses and to thrust out of consciousness anything that clashes with recognised standards of conduct. This process of thrusting out of the mind, initiated by the prohibitions of parents or guardians, becomes habitual, and a mechanism—by which forgetting takes

THEORIES OF THE UNCONSCIOUS

place automatically—is brought into existence. This mechanism is known as the " mechanism of repression."

Since repression begins very early, the unconscious must not be conceived of as consisting merely of *forgotten* experiences, *i.e.*, of experiences once present in consciousness and later thrust into the unconscious. Some of Freud's critics do not seem to understand this. Maurice Nicoll tells us, in referring to Freud's theory, that " the unconscious part of the human psyche contained only what had once belonged to the conscious personal life," * and even Mr Bertrand Russell makes the following statement : " It is not necessary to suppose, as Freud seems to do, that every unconscious wish was once conscious and was then, in his terminology, ' repressed,' because we disapproved of it." † The opposite of this is implied in Freud's theory, and on more than one occasion he has explicitly stated the fact that the unconscious contains much that never saw the light of consciousness.‡ Probably the term " repressed " is misleading, because it seems to suggest a thrusting of conscious material into the unconscious ; but, as Freud explains, it does not matter very much whether we thrust an objectionable person out of our home who has found his way in, or keep him out from the first, shutting the door against him. At any rate Freud regards the unconscious as consisting of experiences that have been repressed out of consciousness because of their painful character, and instinctive strivings that, by the mechanism of repression, have been kept in an unconscious state from the first.

What is the characteristic of these painful impulses that render them subject to the forces of repression and keep them in the unconscious ? And how do repressed emotional experiences lead to mental trouble,

* *British Journal of Psychology*, Vol. IX., p. 230.
† *The Analysis of Mind*, p. 38.
‡ See *Introductory Lectures on Psycho-Analysis*, p. 287.

and the various aberrations which Freud has connected with them ? This leads us to Freud's account of the instinctive life of childhood and the possibilities open to it in the course of its development. Two sets of instinctive impulses are taken into account by Freud— the sexual and the ego impulses. His system proceeds on the assumption that early in life these become quite antagonistic to, and incompatible with, each other. The conflict through which repression takes place depends on the way in which these two sets of tendencies oppose each other. While both types of instinct are recognised, however, Freud regards the sexual ones as fundamental, and his whole theory is built up on this belief. We shall now give a brief account of his theory of the sexual type of instinct.

According to Freud the sexual instincts do not come into existence at the age of puberty ; they are present and operate in every individual from infancy. It is this part of Freud's psychology that has aroused the greatest antagonism. Later we shall contend that much of this antagonism is based on a misconception of Freud's position and use of terms. Here we will content ourselves by pointing out the unreasonableness of the view that the instincts known as sexual could come suddenly into operation at puberty unless they were present in some form, at some level of development, before adolescence. There is a great difference between sexuality as commonly conceived and the type of sexuality characteristic of childhood, out of which the former develops. Freud's view is that the sexual instincts proper are developed out of certain partial trends, organised as opposites, that are found in all childhood. These are sadism and masochism, observationism and exhibitionism. Also certain zones of the body are capable, when stimulated, of producing sensations that are sexually toned.

Sadism (from Count de Sade, whose novels exploit

cruelty of man to woman) signifies the sort of pleasure derived from inflicting pain on others. This tendency to be cruel manifests itself early in children. They take pleasure as a rule in torturing small animals and subjecting them to a lingering death. This pleasure Freud regards as sexual in nature.

Masochism (from L. von Sacher-Masoch, an Austrian novelist, who depicts this form of cruelty practised upon oneself) stands for the pleasure often derived in suffering. It is the passive opposite of sadism.

Observationism is the active pleasure of looking—the tendency "to peep." It means curiosity of a sexual kind, and it inspires many of the awkward questions which the child of five or six asks—especially about the birth of younger children.

Exhibitionism, again, is the opposite of this. It stands for the passive pleasure of being looked at. It represents the tendency of children to "show off." All these traits, whether we agree to characterise them as sexual or not, are certainly to be found in connection with the behaviour of all children.

The zones of the body that are capable of yielding, when stimulated, a sexually toned pleasure are called by Freud "erogenous zones." Not only are the excretory regions and the mouth so characterised, but recently Freud suggests that for aught we know there may be internal erogenous zones as well. The process of deriving pleasure from these sensitive bodily regions is called "auto-eroticism," and it begins very early in the life of the child. The pleasure derived from sucking is sexually toned, and this is the earliest pleasure the child experiences of an erotic kind.

Freud sums up these various types of infantile behaviour, sadistic, masochistic, observationistic, exhibitionistic, and the auto-erotic activity as the expressions of "libido"—a term which in Freud's theory signifies the conative force behind all types of sexual desire. Some analysts call it sexual hunger. Dr Putnam employs the term sexual craving as the most appropriate.

What is the ultimate fate of the libido in the process of its development? This is an important question, for on the transformation of the libido depends the possibility of mental health or illness.

It is a strange conception underlying psycho-analysis that the libido has to be quantitatively as well as qualitatively regarded. It is compared by Freud to a stream, part of which can get divided off from the main channel and utilised for other purposes ; but this conception is essential to his theory, for the quantity of libido to be disposed of, as well as emotional shock and strain, is a factor in the development of neuroses. Normally part of the libido underlying the activities of early life and denoted as sexual goes to the development of the sexual instincts proper ; the other part gets utilised in other ways that are of value to the higher interests of life. It is made to subserve the welfare of the individual and society. The sadistic trend, for example, if it is pronounced in any child, will go in part to the formation of the sexual instincts and in part to useful activities of life, such as are connected with the work of the butcher or the profession of the physician. In exhibitionism the transformation of part of the libido not sexually utilised can be clearly traced in the powers of the orator, preacher, actor, and painter. It is not quite so easy to discover the fate of the libido expressed in the other trends ; but it may be that the explanation of the martyr's joy depends on an excessive masochism, and observationism may lead in the life of the adult to a thirst for knowledge and to researches of various kinds. The process by which the libido becomes transformed and utilised in connection with higher products is known as *sublimation*, and the activities in which it is employed are called " sublimated activities."

It is a misunderstanding of Freud's theory of sublimation to regard the higher activities only as products of the libido and, therefore, as manifestations of the sexual instincts. All that the theory of sublimation involves is that the libido which is not utilised in the development of the sexual instincts proper is utilised by, and reinforces, the higher mental, æsthetic, social, and religious activities. Dr Putnam, in his addresses on psycho-analysis, explains that so far as the sexual instincts are concerned the higher activities exist in their own right, though, in accordance with the theory of evolution, they must be regarded as the products of cruder forms of activity. He argues, as I think correctly, and psycho-analysts do not disagree with him, that in the earlier stages of human life these activities were foreshadowed and were potentially present. All men have some conception of an ideal life which influences the development of these higher activities, and, therefore, these activities cannot be entirely the product of sublimation.

Let us now consider the fate of the libido in *abnormal* cases.

When there are aberrations in mental development the libido may take any one of three possible courses, the deciding factors being the relative strength or weakness of the repressing factors, and the amount of libido that has to be utilised. If the repressing force, represented by early training, the force of education, etc., is not sufficiently strong, the libido may continue in its earlier forms. When this is the case certain perversions arise. Many activities that commonly take place in adult life, such as thumb sucking, are mild forms of such perversion ; others of a more pronounced kind are frequently found disguised in cases of neurotic trouble. Sadism may persist in the form of excessive cruelty. We get an illustration in the case of Nero, who is said to have gloated over the persecution of the early Christians. Some psycho-analysts hold that war is the result of a sudden outburst of this early infantile trait that has been kept for years in a state of repression.

The repressing forces may be too strong instead of too weak. Reaction follows where this is the case. Thus if sadism is unduly repressed it may lead to the type of reaction exemplified in the anti-vivisection movement, or extreme sensitiveness in various forms.

There is another possibility: the repressing force may neither be too strong nor too weak—the libidinous tendencies may be quite as strong as the repressing factors so that neither of the opposing tendencies will win in the conflict. It is on conditions of this kind that the neurotic trouble depends. Every neurotic trouble is a symptom in which a compromise between the repressing and repressed factors is involved. On the one hand, the neurosis represents the breaking forth of unconscious tendencies into consciousness; on the other hand, the disguised form in which they appear, and the pain they cause to the individual are means of satisfying the repressing factors. Thus every neurosis is a compromise formation resulting from an unsuccessful unconscious conflict.

So far we have represented psycho-analysis in its earlier stages, and most expositions of the subject that we have read do not advance further. They are entirely taken up with the description of the conflict that takes place between the libidinous and egoistic impulses, the latter being connected with the moral, social, and religious standards of society. In recent years, Freud has developed another conception to which he attaches the greatest importance, and according to which he is able to explain not only the development of neurotic trouble, but the specific form the trouble may take in any particular case. The clearest statement of this new advance is given in the following utterance of Freud himself : " We have had good grounds for inferring that at the beginning of individual development all libido is attached to one's own person ; as we say, it ' engages ' one. It is only later that, in conjunction with the satisfaction of the main natural functions, the libido reaches out from the ego to external objects, and it is not till then that we are able to recognise the libidinous impulses as such and to distinguish them from the ego impulses. The libido can be later released from its attachment to these objects and again withdrawn into the ego. The state in which the libido is bound up with the ego we call Narcissism, after the Greek myth of the young Narcissus who was in love with his own image.

"We thus regard the course of individual development as an advance from Narcissism to object-love, but we do not believe that the whole libido ever passes over from the ego to the objects of the outer world. A certain amount of it always remains bound to the ego, so that Narcissism survives in a certain degree even when object-love is highly developed. The ego is a great reservoir out of which the libido streams towards its destined objects and into which it flows back again from these objects The ' object-libido ' was, to begin with, ' ego-libido,' and may become so again. For complete health it is necessary that the libido should retain its full mobility. In picturing this reciprocal relationship between love of others and self-love we may think of an amœba, whose protoplasma sends out pseudopodia, projections into which the substance of the body pours, but which can at any time be again retracted so that the form of the protoplasmic mass is once more restored." *

It is clear that according to this theory the fate or

* *The International Journal of Psycho-Analysis*, Vol. I., p. 19.

disposal of the libido in the course of life must be conceived of in a new way. We shall now look at the matter from this later point of view. The life history of the libido may be traced not so much according to its manifestations as according to the objects to which it gets attached. At first, as we have seen, the infant derives all erotic pleasure from itself, especially from the " erogenous zones." At this stage the libido is wholly directed towards the self. Observation of the behaviour of children will bear this out. They reveal a number of traits, which, if they were found amongst adults, would remind one of the megalomaniacal delusions of certain forms of insanity. These are especially the sense of self-importance and the ego-centric attitude towards the world. This is called " primary Narcissism," to distinguish it from the neuroses that later develop by a return of the Narcissism to the infantile level. When primary Narcissism is abandoned the libido generally gets attached to the parents or to those who have to do with the care of the child. This is the next stage in the development of the libido. One of the parents is usually the first love-object of the child. The boy, as a rule, directs his libido towards the mother and the girl towards the father. In this attitude of the child there exists the possibility of perversion and tragedy in later life. The relation between parents and children is of the greatest importance for the later development of character.

In its further development the libido may get attached to some member of the same sex outside the family circle ; in this way friendships are formed. Or it may get attached to a member of the opposite sex and lead to marriage. Again the libido interest may get connected with some ideal for which alone a man may live, and for which he may be willing to sacrifice much. These ideals, according to the amount of libido which they receive, get " over-valued." Here we have the clue to many forms of prejudice and fanaticism.

The foregoing is a brief indication of the normal course of the libido, according to the objects to which it is directed in the course of mental development. We have now to indicate its fate if turned aside from its proper channel. In this case two possibilities are open. First, instead of the libido passing through its various stages of development from one object to another, it may remain " fixed " at some infantile level. When this occurs we have mental abnormalities of various types, according to the condition of each individual life, temperament, training, environment, etc. The fixation of the libido at any one of the early stages, which it usually traverses in the course of normal development, explains those cases of mental disorder to which an individual has always been subject. While in body the child has developed in the course of life, in mind—at least in some of its aspects— no such development has taken place. What is quite natural in the child, if continued to adulthood, is regarded as a manifestation of mental disorder. The following unanalysed case has come under my notice. It illustrates how the " fixation " theory accounts for many of the abnormalities with which we are familiar. We shall call the subject Mr B. He is thirty years of age. His father is a successful business man holding a very high and responsible position. Every opportunity of making a success of life was granted to him. He was put to the best local public schools, but always shrank from study and would not remain at school. He was then sent to a local boarding school, where it was thought he would be kept more strictly to his studies and would not have the same opportunity to get away from the control of his teachers ; but this also proved futile since he took advantage of every opportunity to escape and return home. Finally he was sent to a boarding school in England in the hope that distance from home might prove helpful, but to his parents' surprise, at the end of a week, he was at home again. Thus the years of his school life passed.

When fifteen years of age his father thought of putting him into some business. He soon found, however, that the boy was as much averse to business as to school. One form of occupation after another, for which large sums of money were paid as fees, was tried. In every conceivable way the boy was induced to settle down to the task of life that best suited him. Apparently, however, no occupation fitted in with his peculiar mental constitution. He showed a dislike to work of all kinds as though he were incapable of facing " reality." Every attempt he made to adapt himself to life was short-lived, and though now in the prime of manhood, and apparently physically fit, he remains a useless member of society.

The father is of the opinion that all that is wrong with him is extreme laziness; but this is no explanation. It is the laziness that has to be explained, and psycho-analysis helps us to find a solution to cases of this type. I have asked the father some questions about the way in which the boy spends his time. The information received points to the persistence in his case of infantile traits and tendencies. His chief occupation when alone is either that of devising means for the capture of birds, or of reading such exciting stories as entrance children of five or six years of age. His only companions are children, and with them he revels in imaginary battles in which he always fancies himself as the chief of a Red Indian army. Not long ago the battle became somewhat realistic. He formed the boys into two opposing armies. One, the Red Indian army, of which he was chief, was equipped with dangerous weapons—sticks, knives, etc. The result was that serious wounds were inflicted on many members of the imaginary enemy. Recently a detailed scheme of adventure, in which his army was to take a leading part, fell into his father's hands, and it serves to bring out how highly phantastic is the world in which this man lives. All psycho-analysts agree that there is a close analogy between the infantile life of the civilised individual and the life of the race at its low stages of development. In the case we have described there is some evidence for the truth of this. Infantile and pre-civilised mental traits are found side by side.

As the case is unanalysed we cannot say at what level fixation has taken place. Freud regards the occupation of the libido with the mother as the most common form of fixation. He calls fixation at this stage the " œdipus complex," from the legend of the youth Œdipus, who murdered his father and afterwards unwittingly married his mother. His belief is that the œdipus complex is the nuclear complex for all neuroses. Though I have received no information with regard to the relationship in which the young man whose life story we have partially told stands to his mother, yet there are some things that point to this as the possible source of the trouble. The parents decided one day to break up their home, and this they did. The mother went away for a period of six months during which time the father and son lived in lodgings. Strange to relate, the father during this time was able to induce the son to begin work. He continued to work for three months, and throughout this period high hopes were entertained that at last the boy was turning away from phantasy to reality. But the mother returned, and, a couple of weeks later the work was abandoned and the boy lapsed back to his former ways.

The writer has made some effort to analyse this case, but so far all approaches have been resisted, chiefly because of the boy's extreme shyness and unwillingness to meet any stranger. Should analysis become possible the œdipus complex may be found at the root of the trouble.

The " fixation " theory explains those cases in which the libido has gone wrong from the beginning, but there are hysterics whose trouble did not show itself until after the critical years of childhood had been left behind. Mental disorders often develop late in life. Jung brought this point as an objection to Freud's theory in its earlier form, but this difficulty has now been removed by the incorporation of the Narcissistic conception, and the clearer explanation, on the Narcissistic basis, of the mental abnormalities that develop in the course of life. The libido may not only remain fixed to some infantile level, but it may return in later life to the same level. This process is called by Freud " regression." The term has also another meaning, which we shall consider later in this chapter.

The factors that bring about regression may be very varied, but they are all of the nature of a " deprivation." By this is meant that the object with which the flow of libido was connected gets removed or destroyed, and if a suitable substitute object is not found the libido regresses to the infantile levels. De Quincey tells us in his *Confessions* of a narrow escape he once had from being overwhelmed by a river that suddenly began, as it seemed to him, to flow backwards. Something analogous to this takes place when the libido is deprived of its object ; but escape in this case is not so easily managed. Often the mental life is completely destroyed.

On the level which the libido reaches in the course of its regression depends the type of mental trouble which results. The regression may take place to the stage of auto-eroticism. Freud suggests that in the case of hysterical paralysis and anæsthesias the areas affected are usually the " erogenous zones," which in childhood were the source of erotic gratification. If the libido returns to the " Narcissistic " stage trouble of the type of paranoia follows, in which the patient withdraws from reality and becomes excessively ego-centric. The writer knows a man who, when intoxicated, always imagines himself to be Napoleon and spends most of his time admiring himself in the mirror. This is a form of " secondary narcissism." Perversions of all kinds, as well as the different types of hysterical trouble, are explained by the extent of the regressive process. In this respect, as well as in others, psychoanalysis is in advance of other theories. One of the great weaknesses in the theory of Janet we found to be its inadequacy to account for the specific form which mental disorder in any particular case assumed. The theory of Freud satisfactorily fills up this gap.

Before passing on to the next point, we may state in a sentence or two Freud's attitude to the question of heredity as a factor in the causation of mental disease. From the account we have given of his theory it might be concluded that hereditary factors do not count. This, however, is not strictly accurate. Freud admits the influence of heredity in the production of mental trouble, but, as compared with post-natal experiences, he has assigned to it a very insignificant rôle. Of the two types of factors that influence mental development—heredity and environment—the latter is by far the more important. We may come into the world inheriting certain predispositions, but these are of little consequence as compared with the dispositions that are developed in early life. The stages which the libido leaves behind in the course of its development may be viewed as dispositions that continue to influence the conscious life, and to which the libido easily regresses when deprived of its proper object. These dispositions, resulting from the experiences of early life, form the most important part of the unconscious.

(ii) The probing of the Unconscious—

From the account we have given of the psychoanalytic theory it will be quite plain that the seat of mental trouble, in at least many of its forms, is in the unconscious. The question, therefore, naturally arises —by what means do psycho-analysts reach the unconscious and restore the memories and feelings of early days, that in their repressed condition have been causing trouble ? This question we shall now answer briefly. In psycho-therapeutic methods, other than psycho-analysis, hypnosis is usually resorted to as the means of getting at the unconscious. The New Nancy School, as we have seen, does not advocate hypnosis in its deeper forms, but for the most part this is the method adopted by those physicians of the mind who are not psycho-analysts. Freud himself has no use for hypnosis, though other psycho-analysts have not entirely abandoned it. He has substituted another method of exploring the unconscious and bringing its contents to light.

This method is known as that of " free association," and it is made use of in two forms. In the first place, the patient is asked to express quite freely all the random thoughts that come into his mind. He is counselled not to hesitate to give expression to an idea because it seems ridiculous, or trivial, or even painful. Every effort to inhibit ideas must be abandoned, and the critical faculty must be completely suspended. The influence of suggestion on the production of ideas must be carefully guarded against. For this purpose the subject is often asked to close his eyes, to turn his back on the analyst, and to remain as motionless as possible. If all these conditions are present the ideas that float into the mind will be found to originate in the unconscious, and the skilled interpreter will, after a number of sittings, be able to track down, by following the associations which the ideas give, the trouble to its source. When the painful memory is brought back to the consciousness of the patient, with its emotional accompaniment, recovery sets in. Breuer's patient, referred to at the beginning of this chapter, upon whom this method was first tried, designated it the " talking cure." This was a unique way of restoring mental health. Instead of writing out prescriptions, as the orthodox physician generally does, the patient was encouraged to talk, and by the ideas that were freely expressed a clue was found to the unconscious source of the trouble.

It is by the interpretation of dreams, however, rather than by any other means, that Freud and his followers endeavour to reach the unconscious ; but in this method " free association " is a constant requisite. Dreams, Freud tells us, are the royal road to the unconscious. There is no element in the dream that is not of some significance. It is a manifestation of some unconscious wish. *The dream is a wish-fulfilment.* The problem is how to account for dreams that obviously are not wish-fulfilments. Most dreams as they are remembered are trivial, incoherent, and absurd. In spite of this Freud tell us they are wish-fulfilments. The characteristics of triviality, etc., are only devices to hide the true nature of the wish which is always repugnant to consciousness. A clear distinction must, therefore, be drawn between the " manifest content " of the dream—the dream as remembered—and the " latent content "—the real meaning of the dream when interpreted. The way in which the latent content is transformed into the manifest content is called the *dream work*. It consists of a fourfold process. First, *condensation*. Many ideas, having little connection with one another in waking life, may be condensed into a single element in the dream. When a single dream element is analysed a whole cluster of ideas may be found represented in it. It is difficult indeed to know when one has exhausted in analysis all that the dream element contains. A second stage in the dream work is known as *displacement*. Often the strangeness of the dream is due to the fact that what is trivial in waking life is peculiarly vivid and prominent in the dream. This is an unconscious method of disguising the real meaning of the dream. The " affect " is withdrawn from the most important dream element and gets transferred to some element of little significance. This is why the most seemingly trivial incident or element in the dream often furnishes the analyst with the clue to the real motive of the dream. *Dramatisation* is the third aspect of the dream work. The latent dream-thoughts always find expression by means of a process of dramatisation in which they unroll themselves before the mind of the sleeper. The abstract idea in waking life is set forth in a picturesque, figurative form in the dream, and thus hides from consciousness the dream's real nature. Lastly, in every dream *secondary elaboration* takes place. By this is meant the process by which the dream comes to assume any measure of congruity and coherence. This process is effected more in the stages of semi-consciousness when, awaking from the dream, the attempt is being made to recall its details, than during the dream state.

Other factors in the dream we shall consider in the next section, but from what has been stated it will be obvious that the dream stands in the same relation to the unconscious of the normal individual as the hysterical symptom does to that of the abnormal. The dream is a disguised fulfilment of an unconscious wish. During the waking life the repressing forces (called by Freud the *censor*) prevent the unconscious from reaching consciousness ; but at night " the censor " is partly off guard, and by disguising itself the unconscious can elude him and enter unnoticed into consciousness. Freud regards the dream thought of the normal as closely resembling the mental processes of the hysteric, and it is on this account, as well as on account of the fact that the dream is " the royal road to the unconscious," that Freud has attached such immense importance to dream interpretation. Now, in connection with the analysis of dreams, free association is constantly made use of. Some of the dream symbols are regarded by psycho-analysts as having constant meanings, so that whenever they are met with in the dream they receive without further ado the meaning with which they are connected. This is disputed, however, by some analysts who argue that every symbol in the dream depends on the past history of the dreamer, and must receive careful analysis.

The procedure in analysing dreams is as follows. The patient, having recited the dream, is asked by the physician to give associations to its various elements. Whatever ideas are first suggested to the mind, as it is turned to any part of the dream, are to be freely expressed. In this way some long-forgotten experience is often recalled to consciousness, and the subject is always mentally relieved as a consequence.

In addition to the method of free association and the analysis of dreams, the method of *word-association tests* is also used as a means of probing the unconscious. Jung discovered this method and has devoted a large work to its exposition, but the followers of Freud speak of it as an adjunct, rather than as essential to psychoanalysis. It is useful when dreams are not available for analysis ; otherwise its use is not encouraged. Those who are not Freudians in the strict sense have in recent years—especially in cases of war neuroses—employed this method with great success.

The physician or analyst in adopting word-association begins by preparing a list of carefully chosen words. Jung has a list of one hundred words, which in the course of his experiments he has found most useful. As each word is called out by the analyst the subject is asked to respond by the first idea that enters his mind. The word given by the doctor is called the stimulus word, that by which the patient responds is known as the reaction word, while the time that elapses between the stimulus and reaction words (usually measured by means of a stop-watch) is called the reaction time. Usually the patient responds to the stimulus word without hesitation. Thus, if the doctor calls out the word " ship " the patient may reply at once with the word " ocean "—the reaction word being associated somehow with the stimulus word. When, however, a word is called out, and the patient hesitates before a response is given, the presence of an unconscious complex is indicated. This word *complex*, first used by Jung, stands for a group of ideas in the unconscious, which are held together by a peculiar emotional tone or affect. When a stimulus word is uttered that has any associations with the buried complex, emotional disturbance takes place and the patient is unable to respond in the usual reaction time. Once the clue has been discovered the doctor can follow it up with other appropriate stimulus words, until the forgotten disturbing experience is brought into the light of consciousness.

Dr William Brown * gives us the following illustration of the use of this method. A soldier suffering from extreme loss of memory, hysteria, and mental distraction came to him for treatment. In the course of the word-association tests the word " death " was given. The soldier remained silent for twenty seconds and then gave the curiously associated word " geranium." In the course of further tests the specialist discovered that twenty years earlier the patient had known a girl who had been nicknamed " the Geranium Girl," after a cigarette advertisement. He had a very close friend, J, who became engaged to this girl, J had asked the soldier patient, while he himself was at college, to take the girl out to theatres, as she was very lonely. The result was that the girl fell in love with the

* *The British Medical Journal*, December 1920.

soldier, who, however, did not love her in return. On learning the facts, his friend J became very cool towards him and this so upset the patient that he shot himself. He, however, recovered. After a football accident J died suddenly. His friend, the soldier, being ill himself, did not hear of the death, and in mistake was shown into the room where the man lay dead in his coffin.

This led to a terrible mental disturbance, and ultimately loss of memory; but during all the years the memory continued in the unconscious. It was only through the clue given by the word " geranium " that the specialist came upon the cause of the disturbance. The patient afterwards was completely cured. Jung tells us that not only may prolonged reaction time be a " complex indicator," but so also may be unusual modes of reaction, such as a profession of failure to hear or understand the stimulus word, or a repetition on the patient's part of the stimulus word instead of an associated word. This reveals resistance on the part of the patient's unconscious, and whenever resistance takes place an unconscious complex is being approached.

(iii) No account of psycho-analysis is complete without some reference to the relationship between Freud, Jung, and Adler.

Jung was for a time a close disciple of Freud, and the latter admits that he owes much to Jung's expositions of the theory and his efforts to make it known. The time came, however, when Jung could no longer accept in its entirety the Freudian conception, and, especially on the question of sexuality he broke away from his master.

Freud, as we have seen, uses the term libido in the sense of sexual hunger or impulse. Jung uses it in the sense of psychical energy in the broadest sense. The word is very similar in its meaning, when used by Jung, to the conception of " élan vital " in Bergson's philosophy. Both the libido and the " élan vital " are working conceptions. The latter stands for the idea of an original impulse that has been forcing life along divergent channels. Were it not for this impulse, life would have stopped at its simpler forms. It is the fundamental urge of élan vital that forces life into ever more complex forms.

Libido, in the sense in which Jung employs it, signifies a psychic energy in the widest sense, of which the sex impulses are only one manifestation. It may be regarded as the mental counterpart to the conception of energy in physics. It is probably because of the close relationship of this theory with that of Bergson's that Freudians are always inclined to attack Jung's theory as " philosophical," in contrast to the strictly scientific point of view which, as they claim, is characteristic of Freud's theory.

On the basis of this change of meaning in the fundamental conception of the libido, it follows that the theory of neurosis put forth by Jung must differ considerably from that of Freud. Jung's view is that the real source of neurotic trouble is some present difficulty and not the conflicts of early life. The psychic energy in its normal flow comes up against some barrier ; it accumulates as a stream would, whose course was dammed, and if its attempts to break through fail, regression takes place to earlier mental levels. If the individual finds that normal adaptation to reality fails, then more primitive means of adaptation are resorted to. Dr Maurice Nicoll, who is one of Jung's disciples, gives us the following case *. An officer who had been slightly wounded in the arm and had shown symptoms of shock, including slight battle-dreams, was engaged for some months in administrative work connected with a munitions factory. During this period he had no battle-dreams and enjoyed a fair degree of health. His work, however, began to grow difficult. Disagreeable factors of a personal nature began to appear. Coincidently with

* *Lancet*, June 1918.

this he began to have battle-dreams again, and other symptoms reappeared. This case shows a slight degree of regression in the presence of a difficult situation, causing the revival of recent emotional experiences. Usually in the case of neurotic trouble retreat from reality goes much further, and the patient adopts the infantile modes of adaptation to life.

We shall devote a section to Jung's theory at a later stage of this chapter, and also offer whatever comments on it may seem relevant. So we may now consider briefly the theory of Adler in relation to that of Freud. Adler was also a disciple of Freud and he has diverged from his master to an even greater extent than Jung.

The basis of mental trouble, according to Adler, is an " inferiority complex." When an individual suffers from organic defect a feeling of inferiority takes place. The individual strives against this and endeavours to bring about compensations. This explains those classical cases, such as that of Demosthenes, who began with a speech defect and ultimately became the famous orator of Greece. When the efforts at compensation fail, then mental conflict ensues with its varied train of nervous ills. Illness is to be viewed, according to this theory, as a means of compensation for organic inferiority where other means of compensation are not available. At first it is not quite clear how falling into illness can be regarded as compensatory. Neuroses, however, serve to obtain one thing that otherwise could not be secured, viz., the attention of others. As Jung puts it, " there is no better means of tyrannising over a whole household than by a striking neurosis. Heart attacks, choking fits, convulsions of all kinds achieve enormous effects that can hardly be surpassed. Picture the fountains of pity let loose, . . . the hurried running to and fro of the servants, . . . and there in the midst of all the uproar lies the innocent sufferer to whom the whole household is even overflowingly grateful, when he has recovered from the spasms." *

Adler's theory may be regarded as the opposite of Freud's. It takes into account the ego impulses only, and aims not at supplementing but at supplanting the Freudian theory. Adler has even dropped the title " Psycho-analysis " and adopted that of " Individual Psychology." There can be no doubt that the feeling of inferiority and the effort to compensate for it play a large part in human life, and Adler's system, therefore, contains much that is valuable. We believe, however, that Freud's criticism of it is just : " The picture one derives from Adler's system is founded entirely upon the impulse of aggression. It has no place at all for love." †

From the standpoint of the unconscious Adler's theory is not nearly so important as that of Freud or Jung. The sense of inferiority is described as half-conscious and very little is made of the unconscious. This being the case, it is not necessary to pursue our investigations of Adler's views further. Let us turn rather to a more detailed consideration of the theories of the unconscious held by Freud and Jung, adding an account of yet another theory held by Dr W. H. R. Rivers.

II

TYPES OF UNCONSCIOUS THEORIES

(i) The Theory of Freud—

In the final chapter on " The Interpretation of Dreams " Freud sums up his general account of the mind and its processes. He makes it plain that he gives us no preconceived theory, but one that was suggested by the study of normal and abnormal mental

---

* *Papers on Analytical Psychology*, pp. 389-390.
† *International Journal of Psycho-Analysis*, Vol. I., p. 305.

states. This, in my opinion, is the great merit of Freud's theory—*it is based on facts* and endeavours to be true to them.

The mind is divided by Freud into two parts—the conscious and the unconscious. His account of consciousness is very simple. It consists of all those mental processes of which at any moment we are aware. The word *awareness* gives us the key to the meaning of consciousness as he conceives it. He does not concern himself with such phrases as the "fringe of consciousness" or the "threshold of consciousness," neither does he analyse the constituents of consciousness. We are not told whether consciousness consists of thinking, feeling, and willing, and there is no distinction drawn between consciousness and self-consciousness; consciousness is simply awareness.

Two attributes of consciousness as thus defined are, however, emphasised by Freud. First, *it is a selective agency*. It exercises the power of choice. It is teleological or purposive, and its selective function is based on the pleasure-pain principle. Consciousness tends to select pleasurable experiences and reject those that are painful. Bergson describes consciousness in the same way; he attributes to it selective power and defines it as "the organ of attention to life," but he does not base this function of consciousness on the pleasure-pain principle so much as on the principle of utility. Myers, as we have seen, characterises consciousness in the same way; it is "a function adapted to earth life." Freud recognises the reality principle and admits that the ego-instincts conform to it, but he holds that the reality principle is only a modification of the pleasure principle. To this point we shall again return in subsequent pages.

The second point about consciousness is regarded by Freudians as quite original and of great importance. *Freud compares consciousness to a sense organ*, the function of which is not merely the reception of impressions from the external world, but also and chiefly the perception of the subjective, psychical processes. These processes go on all the time, and it is the function of consciousness to make us aware of them, and differentiate their qualities.

The psychical processes that take place when we are not aware of them form the unconscious. Freud has, therefore, no more difficulty in believing in the existence of unconscious processes than he has in believing in the existence of objects in the external world when they are out of sight. All the time these processes are going on, the end-product of which alone appears in consciousness. A favourite metaphor employed by Freudians in explaining Freud's psychology of the unconscious is that of the factory. Conscious mental processes may be compared to the articles in a shop window, about the manufacture of which from raw materials the average spectator knows nothing, though the articles would never be there unless a whole series of complicated processes had been previously carried out. In the same way processes take place in the factory of the unconscious of which the average individual knows nothing. He can only perceive the thoughts, etc., in the window of consciousness, but these only represent the end-products of the hidden mental processes. The analogy goes further for, as everyone knows, the end-products only represent a fraction of what is produced in the unconscious. There is far more in the unconscious than appears as conscious processes. Further, as the goods produced in a factory may influence our conduct in life without our knowledge of their existence, so unconscious mental processes can affect our lives without our being in any way cognisant of them.

The unconscious also is a storehouse of our memories. It contains the whole of our life's history. No experience through which we pass is ever wholly lost. It remains throughout the years in some form in the unconscious.

There is, of course, nothing new in this latter point. Long before the days of Freud the influences of past experiences on the subsequent history of the individual were recognised. There is, in fact, no theory of the unconscious since that of Leibniz in which this point is ignored. It may, however, be claimed for Freud that he assigns a far greater importance to the influence of the past personal history than do preceding writers. It is to be noted at the same time that another present-day writer, Bergson, has carried the idea at least as far as Freud. The element of importance in this point in the Freudian theory is the emphasis laid on what happens in the very early years of life. It is the first five years that, according to Freud, mean the most for the subsequent life. Upon the trends and habits then formed depend the weal or woe of the individual.

Let us now consider what exactly may be claimed as original in Freud's theory of the unconscious.

(a) Reference ought to be made at first to Freud's twofold division of the unconscious and the terminology employed. We found hints in earlier writers of a difference in the contents of the unconscious, but Freud rendered this point very explicit, and used special nomenclature to express it. The unconscious is divided by him into the fore-conscious or pre-conscious and the unconscious proper.

The fore-conscious signifies all those mental states of which at any moment we are unaware, but which may be brought into consciousness without artificial aid, such as hypnotism or the psycho-analytic method affords. This does not mean that fore-conscious ideas can always be easily recalled. It often happens that the attempt to recover a familiar name does not meet with success. The probable explanation is that for the time being it is connected with some complex in the Freudian unconscious. The main characteristic of the pre-conscious is not that it can be *easily* resuscitated, but that it can enter consciousness in *undisguised* form. Nothing incompatible exists between the fore-conscious and consciousness such as would render the passage from one to the other difficult or impossible. The pre-conscious, therefore, may be defined as consisting in those mental states that are outside consciousness, but which are never inaccessible to consciousness in undisguised form. Freud holds that every experience of life may be discovered later in the pre-conscious. It does not follow that everything in the fore-conscious enters sometime into consciousness. On the contrary, many experiences of life are never recalled. Bergson suggests that only those experiences of life that are useful to the individual are reproduced ; the trivial and the irrelevant are kept in a suppressed state, because their obtrusion into consciousness would be highly embarrassing. Presently we shall have something further to say on this question.

The unconscious proper represents the more important part of Freud's theory. Roughly speaking, the pre-conscious is the unconscious of orthodox psychology. It is in the unconscious as defined by Freud that we get his distinctive contribution to the subject. Unlike the fore-conscious the chief characteristic of the un-conscious is its incompatibility with conscious standards, and its consequent failure to enter con-sciousness, except in a disguised or symbolical way. Already in the first section this was made clear. Here our intention is to deal with the point more in detail. The general differentiating mark of the unconscious is its incompatibility with consciousness ; but of what nature is this incompatibility ? Why must the un-conscious become disguised before it can be received into consciousness ? Freud's reply is—*by reason of its painful character.* The unconscious consists of primitive, infantile experiences and impulses that are incompatible with the standards of later life and so are kept out of consciousness. Between the unconscious and consciousness a barrier is set up which functions in a threefold way.

1. It constitutes a repressing force keeping the unconscious from entering consciousness. Freud compares the unconscious to the Titans in the ancient myth who, because they rebelled against the gods, were cast into Tartarus. Huge mountains were rolled upon them, the weight of which kept them in the underworld. They could never become restored to their former position, though periodically they sought to rebel against their enforced position and caused the mountains to shake and tremble. The mountains in the myth stand for the repressing forces in the Freudian psychology. These forces are constituted by the social conventions, the moral standards, the religious teaching of the time. We seek to bring our life into conformity with these, but the conformity is only outward and superficial. The old, crude, ego-centric traits remain in a repressed form. Civilisation is but a veneer. It has not abolished the primitive modes of behaviour, and these are liable to affect life in all sorts of subtle ways—and sometimes to break out in fury as in the case of war.

2. The barrier acts also as a defence against attempts from without to enter consciousness. It not only functions as a repressing force, but also as a mechanism of " resistance." This force is met with in the actual work of psycho-analysis. Whether the method employed is free-association, dream-interpretation, or word-association tests, when the analyst is approaching the unconscious painful complex he meets with resistance on the part of the patient. The form of the resistance often varies. The patient may remain

silent and give no further associations, he may pretend to be confused and ask that the question or word of the analyst be repeated, or he may break into a passion, bitterly attack the doctor and refuse another sitting. When the barrier begins to act as a resisting force the crucial stage of the psycho-analysis is reached, and if the resistance can be broken down there is little difficulty in reaching the unconscious complex.

3. The barrier further acts as a sort of censorship of the unconscious. Already we have noted that the unconscious is ever striving to enter consciousness, but because of its incompatibility with conscious standards it cannot do so in its real nature. If, however, the unconscious is stripped of those features that make it repugnant to consciousness it may then be received by the latter. It is the work of the censor to see that only in a form acceptable to consciousness can the unconscious contents pass through the barrier. The censor in Freud's psychology acts as the editor who will not allow the unvarnished truth to appear in his paper if it is calculated to offend his readers. He, therefore, eliminates the disagreeable passages and returns the article to the writer. The author now rewrites it and presents it again, with the painful truth cloaked in such a way as not to be recognised for what it really is. In this form the editor agrees to its publication. In the same way the Freudian censor will not permit ideas of a painful character to enter consciousness except in symbolical form, and even then only on certain conditions can the unconscious pass the censor. It does so usually in dreams, for in sleep the censor is partly off his guard and the unconscious can, if properly disguised, enter consciousness unnoticed. The fact that dreams are so quickly forgotten by the waking consciousness is explained as due to the activity of the censor, who, on becoming fully aware of what has happened, forces back again the contents of the uncon-

scious that have passed unrecognised into consciousness. The censorship in Freud's system is in many
respects a strange conception. It leads to a considerable amount of personification, since we cannot conceive of a censor who does nothing. It must be
remembered, however, that the conception is only
figurative. It is simply a symbolical way of stating
the inherent incompatibility between the conscious and
unconscious contents.

Recently in Freud's attempt to develop a " metapsychology " he has brought out, much more fully than
he had done previously, the difference between the
various departments of mental life—conscious, fore-
conscious, and unconscious. Every mental process
must be looked at from three points of view, which he
calls topographical, economic, and dynamic. We shall
refer to the economic and dynamic characteristics of
mental processes presently. In dealing with the topography of the mind he is only stating more fully than
he had done the fact that, not only may the mind be
divided into systems, but we may know what are
the characteristics of any process by the system in
which it takes place. Thus he states that processes
occurring in the unconscious are incapable of mutual
contradiction, possess no idea of negation, have no
relation to time or external reality, are governed by
the pleasure principle, and undergo condensation and
displacement with absolute freedom.

(b) *The two Mental Systems:*

Another important characteristic of the teaching of
Freud is his conception of the primary and secondary
psychic systems that form the precursors of the unconscious and pre-conscious respectively. He thinks of the
mind as a mental apparatus with a sensory and motor
end and capable of receiving stimuli from within and
without. These stimuli set up excitations at the
sensory end, and these discharge themselves at the

motor end. The fact that a movement is set up in the apparatus indicates that energy is involved. This energy is generally called by psycho-analysts " affect." A certain amount of this affect is attached to every complex, and the amount of energy varies according to the nature of the ideas involved. Some ideas are invested with far more affect than others, as everyone can easily verify.

One consideration of great importance about this psychic energy is its capacity for " displacement." The affect attached to one idea or group of ideas can become dissociated and invested in another idea resembling it in some respect. This process of displacement usually goes on in the unconscious, and it does so with great readiness—no form of association being too narrow a bridge to allow of the passage from one idea to another. In the explanation of neuroses the mechanism of displacement has been of great service. It accounts for the attitude of the person who is afraid of perfectly harmless things, such as closed doors or tunnels. The affect connected with a group of painful ideas, or unpleasant experiences, has become repressed and has then been attached to external objects that have some slight connection with the repressed complex. In reality the neurotic does not fear the object which he seems to fear. What he really fears, as Dr Putnam so often says, is himself.

Unconscious displacement of affect also accounts for much in normal mental functioning. It probably underlies the spinster's love of pets, and also much of the fanaticism and prejudice that commonly exist. The repressed affect may become attached to any idea in the fore-conscious and in this way some ideas are " overvalued "—they receive affect out of all proportion to their worth. In dreams, as we have already seen, we repeatedly get proof of this. Some part of the pre-conscious contents, that result from the thought of the preceding day, is frequently used in the dream, but these are charged with an amount of energy in the dream state that render them far more vivid than they appeared to be in waking life. Freud's opinion is that every dream originates in the unconscious; it is the fulfilment of an unconscious wish, and it uses the fore-conscious material as its language.

In the first section of this chapter reference was made to the idea of " regression " in the Freudian theory. One meaning of the term was given ; the second comes now into view. A stimulus acting at the sensory end of the apparatus sets up a movement that normally discharges itself at the motor end. Sometimes, however, as in sleep, the motor end gets closed down, and excitations arising from internal or external stimuli move back towards the sensory end, where they produce hallucinatory experiences. Regression in its second meaning, therefore, stands for that process by which a need that is normally met by an appropriate movement receives gratification in hallucinatory experiences.

Another point about the psychical energy is that excessive accumulation of it results in a tension which is perceived as discomfort until discharge takes place. This discharge is experienced as pleasure or gratification. In the primary system, which is the basis of the unconscious, a need—say, the need of the child for food —gives rise to a desire to reproduce the memory of a previous satisfaction of the need, and for a time this hallucinatory experience brings a measure of relief. The gratification, however, received in this way is but short-lived, the tension returns and increases, after which new mental processes are put into operation, the effect of which is to modify the environment, e.g., in the case of the child, to secure food. The mechanism by which this is brought about is the secondary system.

In the primary system the freest possible movement

takes place, the characteristics of logical thought are lacking, the affect " radiates " over a great variety of ideas, the faintest resemblance between them being a sufficient link of association. The secondary system comes into operation as an inhibitory force to this freedom of movement on the part of the primary system.

Two services are rendered by the secondary system : first, *an economic one*. The primary system with its freedom of movement tends to expend too much energy without useful results. The secondary system by controlling the movement brings about an economy of energy, and better results follow. This is the second point of view from which, according to Freud's " metapsychology," a mental process can be examined. " By an economic point of view Freud means one in which the attempt is made to ascertain the laws covering the production, distribution, and consumption of definite quantities of physical excitation or energy according to the economic principle of the greatest advantage with the least effort." * The second service has to do with the *pleasure-pain principle*. The primary system is constantly striving for pleasure ; it can only wish and imagine the fulfilment of wishes. Now certain of these strivings for pleasure are inhibited by the secondary system, because they are incompatible with the conscious standards set up by moral, social, or religious tradition. Thus we have in the activity of the secondary system the prototype of what in later life would be termed repression.

(c) One other characteristic of Freud's theory needs emphasis. He tells us that we can look at a mental process from the dynamical point of view as well as from that of topography or economics, and the unconscious, according to Freud, is essentially dynamical. Freudians claim this to be a leading distinction between

* *International Journal of Psycho-Analysis*, Vol. I., p. 175.

the theory of their master and those of early writers. Pre-Freudian theories are often called "limbo" theories. The unconscious is conceived merely as a storehouse and not as a factory. After our study of the early theories, such a claim cannot be regarded as representing the whole truth. We had active conceptions of the unconscious presented in Kant, Schopenhauer, and Hartmann, and less clearly in Herbart and others. At the same time it must be maintained that Freud goes much further in emphasising this point than do earlier writers. From the brief account already given of the history of the libido in its courses of development, of the mechanisms of displacement, resistance, censorship, etc., this fact cannot but be admitted. Indeed, the impression that a reading of Freud's psychology creates is that for him the meaning of symptoms, dreams, everyday mistakes, etc., is not nearly so important as the underlying forces by which their existence is explained.

One or two points, however, are not in my opinion made sufficiently clear. While it is most clearly stated that the unconscious is dynamical, as a matter of fact we hear as much about "unconscious ideas" as we do about "unconscious affects" or "conations." Of course a dynamic view of the unconscious could be maintained if the term "unconscious ideas" was used consistently to explain its contents. Thus Coué deals only with unconscious ideas, but because an idea tends to realise itself, the unconscious is something in which work is going on continually. But this is clearly not the view of Freud, for he speaks of unconscious affects and unconscious strivings or conations. Whether these, together with ideas, are to be found in the unconscious, and, if so, which is the more dominant element, or whether any element can be said to be more important than another, are questions that in my opinion are not made clear by psycho-analysts. Indeed, the literature of the subject is not always free from contradiction on this point. Thus, when dealing with the process of displacement the impression generally conveyed is that the idea from which affect is withdrawn always falls into the unconscious, and the affect becomes attached to a new substitute idea that may be conscious. In dealing with regression the affect is described as flowing backward, and reinvesting ideas in the unconscious from which it had previously been withdrawn. On the other hand, Dr Jones in dealing with repression makes the following statement : " There seems to be a prevailing notion that repression is mainly a question of forgotten ideas, whereas the truth is that the whole problem is one of the affective life. Both the repressing force itself and the mental material that is repressed can most accurately be described in affective terms. The so-called painful idea is really only a sign that represents the whole complex, and when the latter is in a state of repression the idea itself may or may not be inaccessible to consciousness." * On the other hand, in a review of Dr Coriat's recent book entitled *Repressed Emotions*, the reviewer remarks that the title he has chosen for his book does not coincide with psycho-analytical views, for the psycho-analytical theory does not admit the " repression of emotions." †

Probably, when clearly stated, the position is as described by Dr Jones. It is the affect that is repressed and any ideas that are associated with the affect are also liable to be dragged with it into the unconscious.

On this view can best be explained the fact that the mere revival of a forgotten memory at the root of a neurosis does not always lead to relief from the neurotic symptoms. The revival must be accompanied by emotional intensity, by the discharge of the pent up affect. The position, therefore, seems to be that while

* *The British Journal of Psychology*, Vol. VIII., p. 43.
† *International Journal of Psycho-Analysis*, Vol. III., p. 234.

ideas may and do form part of the unconscious, it is the affect that is all-important.

But if the unconscious consists chiefly of affect or feeling, have psycho-analysts any right to claim for it a specially dynamical character ? If it is dynamical, if active processes are going on all the time in the unconscious, would not conations rather than affects be the more appropriate term by which to describe it ? There can, of course, scarcely be affect without striving. Feeling generally leads to action. Also we have to take Freud's quantitative theory of affect into account. He conceives of affect after the fashion of an electric charge. At the same time, the failure to distinguish clearly between affect and conation cannot but be puzzling to the ordinary reader of psycho-analysis.

Before passing away from Freud's theory there are two points which need attention.

1. Readers unfamiliar with the literature of psychoanalysis will take strong exception to Freud's emphasis on the sexual impulses, as the most fundamental in human nature, and to the comparatively slight treatment which other instincts receive at his hands.

This certainly is the first impression that the average reader receives, but when the meaning which Freud assigns to the term sexual is fully understood, his position is not so extreme and unreasonable, and certainly not so unpalatable, as at first one is led to suppose. As to the meaning of the term, let us quote Freud's own words : " Libido is an expression taken from the theory of the emotions. We call by that name the energy (regarded as a quantitative magnitude, though not at present actually mensurable) of those instincts which have to do with all that may be comprised under the word ' love.' The nucleus of what we mean by love naturally consists (and this is what is commonly called love, and what the poet sings of) in sexual love with sexual union as its aim. But we do not separate from

this—what in any case has a share in the name ' love '
—on the one hand, self-love, and on the other, love
for parents and children, friendship and love for
humanity in general, and also devotion to concrete
objects and to abstract ideas. Our justification lies
in the fact that psycho-analytic research has taught us
that all these tendencies are an expression of the same
instinctive activities; in relations between the sexes
these instincts force their way towards sexual union,
but in other circumstances they are diverted from this
aim or are prevented from reaching it, though always
preserving enough of their original nature to keep their
identity recognisable (as in such features as the longing
for proximity, and self-sacrifice)." *

This statement takes from the theory much that may
seem objectionable. At the same time it is questionable
whether the term sexual should have received such an
extension of meaning, and, if it is to be used in this
general sense, whether some other term such as " love "
would not have been more appropriate.

It may be complained against Freud's theory that
the ego instincts do not receive all the attention that
they deserve. Freud admits this, but defends himself
on the ground that in his special investigations it is
the sexual instincts that have been found to be all-
important, and that we know the ego instincts only by
the resistance they offer to analysis. They are found
in opposition to the sexual impulses, and without their
interference the conflict which often leads to neuroses
would not take place. Recently, new light has been
brought to bear on the ego instincts in connection with
the narcissistic theory, and it is shown that just as the
libido passes through stages of development, so also do
the ego instincts. In some the ego is more developed
than in others, according as the forces of education are
brought to bear upon the life. Influenced in this way,

* *Group Psychology and the Analysis of the Ego*, pp. 37, 38.

a " splitting of the ego " gradually takes place, out of which an " ego ideal " is formed. Without this " ego ideal " the infantile manifestations of the libido may be tolerated, and no conflict can take place. If there is a particularly high " ego ideal " consisting of ideals of purity, truthfulness, etc., all tendencies of an infantile character are opposed by it and become repressed. On the basis of this development of the ego, and the difference between the ego and the ego ideal, conscience and the sense of guilt are explained ; and the higher the ideal the greater the sense of self-condemnation for tendencies and activities that fall below it.

Freud is further criticised for taking no account of the herd instincts. These, according to Trotter in his *Instincts of the Herd in Peace and War,* are as fundamental as the two groups which Freud recognises, and from these, not from the ego instincts, proceed the repressive forces and the resistances which psychoanalysts have shown to exist.

Freud, however, has dealt fully with the herd instincts.* He argues that they are not as primary as the instincts of self-preservation and the sexual instinct, for we can find no trace of them in young children. The dread which children experience when left alone is not, as Trotter argues, a manifestation of the herd instincts, but relates rather to the child's mother and is the expression of an unfulfilled desire. That this is so is proved by the fact that the child is not pacified by the sight of any other " member of the herd," but only by the mother. Later supposed manifestations of the herd instincts, when many children congregate in the nursery and school, are similarly dealt with. When a child learns that the parents love the other children as well as himself, and that a hostile attitude towards them on his part cannot be maintained, he then substitutes for the feeling of jealousy and hatred

* See his *Group Psychology and the Analysis of the Ego.*

that of group feeling, and in this way makes sure of equal treatment for all—if he cannot be the favourite then he makes up his mind that no one else will—and so there springs up the " group spirit." More convincing, however, are some general considerations introduced by Freud in his treatment of these instincts. He thinks that the chief characteristic of group psychology is the need of a leader, and that the crowd is held together by libidinal ties that hold between each member of the crowd and the leader, and in consequence of this between the members themselves. So long as these ties hold the self-love of each member ceases to exist, narcissism is limited, and the individual is willing to sacrifice anything for the sake of the leader. This is illustrated in the two staple groups of the army and the church, in which sometimes an ideal is substituted for a personal leader. When panic ensues, what happens is that the libidinal ties binding the members of the crowd to the leader have somehow been broken, consequently the ties binding the members to one another also get severed ; and then the crowd dissolves, and what becomes dominant is the instinct of self-preservation—" every man for himself."

In this way Freud has got rid of the so-called herd instincts. For him they are only manifestations of the sexual instincts, and whether or not he has been quite successful in his argument it cannot be urged by critics of psycho-analysis that he has completely ignored the herd instincts.

We have to add that the method of dividing all the instincts up into the three groups we have mentioned seems wholly unsatisfactory. It is impossible, I think, to find a purely sexual instinct into which elements of the instincts of self-preservation do not enter, and the same may be said of all the other instincts. When this threefold division is employed it ought to be understood only in the most general way. Dr McDougall's simple enumeration of the instincts seems to be much more satisfactory. Freud, himself, recognises the difficulty of maintaining a clear distinction between the sexual and ego instincts, for he says : " In a whole series of cases it looks as if there might also be conflict between various purely sexual impulses ; at bottom, however, this is the same thing, because of the two sexual impulses engaged in a conflict one will always be found consistent with the ego while the other calls forth a protest from the ego." *

2. There seems to be some confusion in the *use of the term repression.*

Dr Jones, who accurately represents Freud, asserts that *all* forgetting is due to repression. This statement is rather sweeping, especially in view of the negative character of the arguments by which he seeks to support it. Thus he tells us that repressed affect tends to become so radiated that we cannot be sure of any idea into which it does not enter by association and, therefore, we cannot prove that all forgetting is not due to repression. He admits that some forgetting may be traced to the utility principle, but that this latter principle depends on the principle of pleasure, that as a matter of fact " the disturbance to consciousness caused by the intrusion of the irrelevant and useless thoughts might, without much exaggeration, be conceived of in terms of the pleasure principle itself as a mild variety of unlust." † He supports his view by a reference to the fact that in philosophy the expression " utilitarian " is tantamount to " hedonic."

Now, that much of our forgetting is due to repression cannot be doubted. The mind naturally tends to turn away from painful experiences. How often we hear the statement from those who know nothing of psychoanalysis—" that is one of those experiences I would

* *Introductory Lectures on Psycho-Analysis*, p. 294.
† *Papers on Psycho-Analysis*, p. 119.

like to forget ! " Much of our forgetting, however, is carried out without conscious effort. There seems to be a mechanism of repression that works apart from any conscious attention. Many of the mistakes of everyday life, *e.g.*, failure to post letters, forgetting an appointment which in reality we did not wish to keep, unwittingly mistaking the hour of the departure of the train when the journey we should have taken has painful associations, are possibly due to repression.

Some may think that their experience lends no support to this view. It is the painful, they say, that they cannot forget. Freudians would reply by saying that they misunderstand the word painful. It is not those painful experiences such as the death of a friend or a disappointment in business that are meant by the word in psycho-analysis, but rather those experiences to which shame is attached and which are repugnant to moral or social standards. Moreover, Freudians would argue that when a painful experience which we would like to forget keeps obtruding itself into consciousness, it may be fairly concluded that it is acting as a substitute for some other experience or group of ideas more painful still.

Not only do we admit that much of our forgetting is due to repression, but also the difficulty of distinguishing sometimes between the pleasure-pain and reality or utilitarian principles. The cropping up of the memories of all sorts of incidents into consciousness would not only be harmful but also painful. Also it is the case that turning away from painful experiences is often useful. Both principles, therefore, cannot always be kept apart. Where this is so, however, it is not necessary to suppose, as Freudians do, that the pleasure principle is the primary and more fundamental one. There is much that points the other way. What originally is aimed at for purposes of utility may later be sought after for the sake of pleasure alone. In this case the utility principle must be regarded as fundamental. Admitting, however, that the two principles cannot always be clearly distinguished, it would be untrue to say they never can. Conceivably there are occasions when it is beneficial to retain the painful in consciousness instead of repressing it and when, on the other hand, it would be useful to thrust from consciousness the pleasurable. Whether this be so or not, to keep the two apart will prevent confusion. Dr Jones, in his attempt to harmonise these principles, suggests the use of two terms, "hedonic repression" and "utilitarian repression." I think this is to confuse the meaning of repression, which is always used by Freud for what has been thrust out of consciousness, or not admitted to it, because of its painful character. The term should continue to bear this meaning if for no other reason than the avoidance of confusion.

It would be more helpful to confine the pleasure principle to the contents of the unconscious, these having been repressed owing to their painful character. Let the utility principle apply to the fore-conscious material and to it alone. The word repression is never used by the Freudian school for that type of forgetting in which the contents of consciousness are simply thrust into the fore-conscious. The word *suppression* ought to be retained for forgetting of this type. Such suppression usually proceeds according to the utility principle. If this distinction is observed then the terms to be used are not "hedonic repression" and "utilitarian repression," but rather "hedonic repression" and "utilitarian suppression," or more briefly, repression and suppression. What we forget through the operation of the former principle forms the "unconscious." What we forget through that of the latter forms the "pre-conscious." Of course, the pre-conscious may later, through association with unconscious material, come under the dominance of repression and sink into the unconscious, but our contention is that *all* forgetting is not due to repression.

(ii) The Theory of Jung—

From our consideration of Freud's theory it will be apparent that he regards the unconscious as coming into existence in the course of personal history. When a child is born into the world he has no unconscious ; when he reaches the age of puberty an unconscious has developed. This unconscious depends on the forms of repression that are early brought to bear on the mind and that inhibit those mental processes that become incompatible with the standards of later life. It is clear from this that Freud lays much greater stress on the power of environment than on that of heredity in influencing the development of the mental and moral life. A man's fate, no matter from what aspect his life is viewed, depends not so much on the inherent tendencies of his nature as the way in which these are dealt with, especially in the first few years of his life.

Jung agrees so far with Freud. He recognises an unconscious that is built up, as Freud describes it, in the course of individual life ; but this he thinks is not sufficient. There is not only an unconscious that is developed out of personal experience, but one that we bring with us, already formed, into life. Jung must, therefore, recognise to a much greater extent than Freud the power of heredity in influencing the course of later life. Let us consider further his views. He defines the unconscious as " the totality of all psychic phenomena that lack the quality of consciousness," and he divides it into the personal and the collective or impersonal unconscious.

(*a*) The Personal Unconscious :

This part of the unconscious consists of all lost memories, and the incompatible thoughts and feelings that become subject to repression. Jung's personal unconscious, therefore, may be said to contain (1) all that is involved in the Freudian fore-conscious ; (2) all that is involved in the Freudian unconscious. The personal unconscious, he says, consists of those experiences " that have been forgotten and repressed." " We emphatically say that the personal unconscious contains all that part of the psyche that is found under the threshold, including subliminal sense perceptions in addition to the repressed material." *

2. It is the second part of Jung's theory—that of the collective unconscious—that we are especially concerned with, since this is Jung's distinctive contribution to the study of the unconscious. His argument against Freud's theory is not that it is invalid, but rather that it is not an adequate account of the facts. If the unconscious is merely a repressed part of the psychic life of the individual, then, Jung argues, it ought to be possible to exhaust its contents and do away with them in analysis. Experience, however, shows that this is not the case, that no matter how far we carry the analysis we still continue to weave our dreams and phantasies. This suggests that the contents of the unconscious are inexhaustible.

Another type of argument used against the adequacy of the Freudian view is that we seem to contain more than we have acquired : " All great art lifts us beyond our conscious scenes, but when the spell is over we lose the vision and wonder at the depths within us." †

If the theory of Jung rested on these negative arguments alone it would be based on a flimsy foundation indeed. The first argument goes on the assumption that the Freudian unconscious contains only the material that was once conscious and became afterwards repressed ; but we have already pointed out that part of its contents

* *Papers on Analytical Psychology*, pp. 438, 446.
† *British Journal of Psychology*, Vol. IX., p. 232.

have never been conscious and that, therefore, it contains more than on the surface seems possible. Besides, since repression is a mechanism or habit that is in constant operation, it seems impossible ever to reach a stage in analysis when all the contents of the unconscious would have been brought to light. Freud himself suggests that theoretically it would be almost impossible to exhaust all the buried associations of a single dream, and that, as a matter of fact, no dream is ever *fully* interpreted.

The second type of argument receives an answer in the principles of Freud's own theory. All great art is the product of sublimated energy.

When, however, we turn away from these criticisms of the Freudian theory to Jung's constructive work, and consider what the collective unconscious means, his theory becomes much more plausible. The collective unconscious contains all those psychical types of reaction and tendencies that are common to the race. Whatever psychical qualities are of regular and uniform occurrence, and have nothing to do with the individual qualities of particular men, are collective unconscious phenomena. According to this definition the contents of the collective unconscious are of two kinds.

First, the collective unconscious is formed out of *instincts*. Instincts are part of the collective unconscious, because they are not acquired in the course of the individual life, but are inherited and are of " regular and uniform occurrence." Man possesses them not only in common with all the members of the race, but with the lower animals as well. Thus the collective unconscious, in one of its aspects, links us not only with primitive human life, but also with our pre-human ancestry. Accordingly, Jung, in explaining neurotic trouble, holds that regression goes much further than Freud will allow. It does not stop at the infantile layers of the unconscious, but returns to the primitive and even pre-human strata that lie deep in the collective unconscious. When higher adaptation to reality fails and the life energy streams back, it is possible that a successful but much lower type of adaptation may take place. " Partial regression from civilised standards to more brutal planes may bring about a successful adjustment, and this we call *regressive adaptation*. By becoming more of a brute, by allowing hate and lust to animate him a man may successfully endure certain aspects of life in the trenches." * Now, no writer—least of all the Freudians —will deny the fact that we come into the world as the possessors of instinctive tendencies that we inherit from our human and pre-human ancestry. James Harvey Robinson in his recent work, *The Mind in the Making*, maintains that at birth we are all uncivilised, that certain of our most essential desires are brutish— " hunger, thirst, the urgency of sleep, sexual longing, blind anger, striking, biting, the tendency to irrational fears and ignominious flight—all these and others make man continuous with the lower animals. . . . If we could trace our human lineage back far enough we should come to a point where our human ancestors had no civilisation and lived a speechless, naked, houseless, fireless and toolless life. They subsisted on raw fruit, berries, insects and such animals as he could strike down, and his mind must have corresponded with his brutish state." † This author finds three layers underlying the minds of civilised man—the animal mind, the savage mind, and the child mind. With this Freudians are in entire agreement. They find a very close resemblance between the savage mind and that of the child, as they also do between these and the mental characteristics of the neurotic and of the dream state of the healthy adult. Each individual

* *Dream Psychology*—Maurice Nicoll, p. 169.
† *The Mind in the Making*, pp. 68, 86.

in the course of life recapitulates the history of the race.

The relation of instinct to the unconscious will concern us again when dealing with the theory of Dr Rivers, and we shall pass away from it now with a two-fold remark : (a) It is not quite plain how instincts can be unconscious at all. It is probably true that behaviour for which we seek to give rational explanations is based on instinctive impulses. The motivation of many of our acts is not always what we claim it to be. The real motives of much of our conduct are thickly veiled from conscious awareness. If this is what Jung intends, then there is perfect agreement so far as this point is concerned between himself and Freud. Thus one of the most highly honoured of Freud's followers tells us that " men are handicapped by passions, longings, personal ambitions, cravings for success and mastery, to a degree of which they are never wholly conscious. Not only a portion of men's acts but all of them derive some colouring from these sources." *

(b) To the extent to which these instinctive impulses are unconscious they belong rather to the personal than to the collective unconscious. Instincts, we must suppose, would be altogether conscious were it not for repression. Already Jung has included repressed psychic material in the contents of the personal unconscious ; instinctive impulses are among such material and it would seem, therefore, that some unconscious contents belong both to the personal and to the impersonal realms of unconscious life. This is rather confusing and unnecessary, and our conclusion is that so far as instinctive tendencies are unconscious they are so as the result of repression, and, consequently, belong to the personal unconscious. The collective unconscious,

* *Human Motives*—J. J. Putnam, Preface, p. 14.

therefore, so far as instincts are concerned, is non-existent.

The second type of material that forms the contents of the collective unconscious Jung describes as " *latent thought-feelings*," " pre-existent forms of apprehension," " congenital conditions of intuition, viz., the archetypes of apperception which are the a priori determining constituents of all experience." * Jung illustrates and supports his theory by a reference to the patient of Maeder's who believed that the world was his picture book. The phantasy of this uneducated patient only differs, Jung thinks, in elaboration and detail from the system of Schopenhauer, who conceived the world as will and idea. The same primordial thought-feeling underlies both the phantasy and the system of Schopenhauer.

Another illustration is drawn from the discovery by Mayer of the law of the conservation of energy. Jung emphasises the fact that it was a discovery and not the result of deliberate thought. It was the outcome of the revival of a dormant primordial image that lay far down in the unconscious. Jung seeks to substantiate this by an appeal to primitive ways of thinking. If the discovery of the law is the result of the revival of a primitive dormant image, then we must expect to find the corresponding image in primitive thought, and Jung's opinion is that we get it in the idea of power that was current in primitive times, especially in primitive religions. These religions, while differing widely, all agree in attributing the world of existing things to some great power as its source, and this power appears under the name soul, spirit, God, physical strength, fertility, influence, curative remedies. In the Old Testament it is seen in the burning bush ; in the New Testament it appears as the outpouring of the Spirit ; in Heraclitus as " the eternally living fire."

* *British Journal of Psychology*, Vol. X., p. 19.

THE UNCONSCIOUS AND PSYCHO-ANALYSIS

This idea of power, so prevalent amongst primitive peoples, is what Jung calls a " dominant " of the collective unconscious, and to its revival is due the idea of energy in Mayer's law.

Whence comes the idea of " conservation " ? From the general ancient belief of the undying nature of the soul, and especially from that form of the belief known as the transmigration of souls.

This image lies in a latent form in the collective unconscious of everyone, and when suitable conditions arise it becomes aroused and enters consciousness in some form. In the case of Mayer it came as the useful discovery of the law of the conservation of energy.

In seeking to estimate the value of this aspect of the collective unconscious there are some things we admit and others that we question or deny. That there are certain archetypes of thought cannot be disputed. Jung states that the world's great philosophers recognised their importance. Thus in Plato's philosophy the archetypes are held to be the models of the real things, and Kant reduced them to the limited number of the categories. Before the writer ever heard of Jung, the question we are discussing presented itself to him when studying the *Meno* of Plato. Socrates, it will be remembered, proceeds to illustrate the doctrine that knowledge is reminiscence by a practical example. He asks Meno to call one of his numerous pages, a perfectly uneducated lad. Showing this boy a square, Socrates elicits from him the correct view that if the side of such a figure were two feet, the figure itself would be four square feet ; likewise, that a square twice as big as this would consist of eight square feet. Then Socrates asks how big the line would be on which the double line would be described, and the boy promptly replies that it would be double the size of the other.

The question is, how did the boy secure the knowledge that enabled him to answer correctly ? He had no opportunity, according to the *Dialogues*, of previous education. The knowledge, therefore, must have been born with him, in a latent condition, and by the cathartic process—made use of to such an extent in psycho-analysis—the latent became part of the contents of consciousness as actual knowledge.

There is, of course, one respect in which the latent knowledge evoked from the mind of the slave differs from the " archetypes " of Jung's theory ; though it is latent it has been acquired by the soul of the slave in some pre-existent state. The inborn knowledge exemplified here is, therefore, comparable to the knowledge we may all acquire in the course of life and forget ; it may be said to exist in a latent fashion and be capable of being reproduced at any time.

Jung's theory of latent collective knowledge goes on the assumption of heredity as psychically applied. We come into the world in the possession of latent knowledge, which, not we, but our ancestors have acquired and passed on to us at birth. All those conditions of cognition that are " uniform and regular," that belong to all the members of the race, those mental qualities that cannot be attributed to education—these all form part of the collective unconscious, which is an inheritance, a racial background of the mind.

There are some considerations that render the collective unconscious in this sense rather dubious, though I should not go so far as to deny it altogether. The facts, it seems to me, are as Jung states them, but his explanation may be questioned, for the following reasons : (1) It is not possible to state with any degree of certainty how much we have inherited and how much acquired. The process of learning begins very early, and even in the case of the slave of Socrates the true opinions evoked may very well have been gained on his entry into this human life. (2) It is possible that the collective phenomena under consideration may be explained on a physiological basis. What we inherit, it may be held, is not certain mental qualities characteristic of the life of our ancestors, but rather such a modification of the nervous system as renders certain types of thinking necessary. Semon's theory of " engrams " would accord fairly well with the facts. He applies his theory, of course, to the question of memory. An " engram " represents the fact that the results of experience get embodied in modifications of the brain and nerves. But he suggests also that these engrams may be inherited. I would not introduce a physiological theory to account for the facts, were it not that it is easier to think of the law of heredity as operating in the sphere of physiology than in that of psychology. (3) Very much of the material used by Jung as illustrations in support of his theory seems to be quite sufficiently accounted for by the personal unconscious. The phantasy of Maeder's patient referred to would be explained by the Freudians as due to repression that was not successful— the phantasy being a compromise symptom. Schopenhauer's system would be explained as due to some extent, at any rate, to sublimated libido, to libido taken up and utilised in higher mental processes. The idea of energy and other kindred concepts Freudians would refer to the unconscious striving of repressed libido, the very nature of which is to create.

Taking these points into account, it does not seem feasible to attach very much importance to Jung's theory of a collective unconscious. If we can dispense with the concept in favour of the more adequate working of the personal unconscious it is all to the good to do so. " Hypotheses should not be unnecessarily multiplied."

There is another point of considerable importance in which Jung's theory differs from that of Freud, viz. : the matter of the *interpretation* of the unconscious, apart from the question whether the unconscious material is to be classified as personal or collective.

Freud interprets the unconscious strictly according to causal principles. Jung goes beyond the causal modes of interpretation and introduces teleological principles as supplementary to those adopted by Freud. He tells us that he adopts a constructive point of view, as distinct from the purely analytic standpoint of the founder of psycho-analysis. The different points of view are best seen in the method of dream interpretation followed by each investigator. Jung as well as Freud regards the dream as the creation of the unconscious, and, therefore, as the symbolic representation of unconscious tendencies, but the symbolism of the dream receives different treatment at the hands of Jung from that given by Freud. The latter writer, as we have seen, reduces the dream elements by analysis to their associations with the individual's infantile impulses. He explains by the reductive method the cause or origin of the dream. Having done this he regards his task as finished. Jung, on the other hand, while not rejecting the causal method, declares that we actually gain very little by it. He compares the reductive method to an analysis of the bricks and mortar that compose a cathedral in order to account for the reason of its existence. To discover the basal elements of the dream is something, but it is not enough. We must ask—What is the purpose of the dream? What is its bearing on the life of the individual and the problems of the present? Dream symbolism, therefore, has not only a causal significance, but a prospective one as well. The dream, when constructively interpreted, may throw light upon the problems of the dreamer's life that may be to him of great practical value. The following dream of the writer may be taken as illustrating these different points of view. Some time ago he dreamt he was

THE UNCONSCIOUS AND PSYCHO-ANALYSIS

taking a train journey. The ticket he received only
brought him to a certain junction on the way to his
destination. Here he was to change trains and get
another ticket to complete his journey. When, however, he approached the booking-office, he found that
he had completely forgotten the name of the place for
which he was bound ; and after a vain attempt to recall
the forgotten name he decided to take a ticket for an
entirely different place.

The next day an attempt was made to interpret this
dream according to the Freudian method. The result
was that a scene of considerable emotional interest, that
occurred many years ago at a railway junction, was
recalled to consciousness. Thinking over this scene,
associations were made with a still earlier experience
in which a certain insuperable difficulty was presented.
The failure to recall in the dream the name of the forgotten station symbolises this difficulty occurring in
early life. It may be possible to carry the analysis
of this dream further, and, according to Freudians, it
would be necessary to do so, but there is no need to
proceed further for our present purpose.

Now, if instead of interpreting this dream according
to the reductive method the prospective or constructive
method were employed, the result would have been
entirely different. Accordingly, an interpretation on
Jung's principles was attempted. The failure to recall
the forgotten name was again naturally looked upon as
symbolising an insuperable difficulty, but in this case
the difficulty was not in the past, but in the present.
Thinking over the matter my mind turned to a difficulty with which I had for some time struggled in vain.
If now I ask what help I may receive in connection
with this difficulty from the other interpretation of the
dream the answer comes—" the difficulty is insuperable,
ignore it and take up some new enterprise or task."

Which of these interpretations is to be preferred is

not easy to decide. There are difficulties in both methods of interpretation, and much dream interpretation of the kind just given may be wide of the mark and quite valueless.

As compared with Freud's interpretation, that of Jung opens the way to all sorts of speculation. Some dream symbols, according to Freud, always stand for the same idea no matter who the dreamer is. Jung denies this and his argument against it seems to me unanswerable. He cites the following dream of one of his patients : " I was going upstairs with my mother and sister. When we reached the top I was told that my sister was soon to have a child." Now, according to Freud, going upstairs always has a sexual significance. But Jung asks—" If I say that the stairs are a symbol, whence do I obtain the right to regard the mother, the sister, and the child as concrete ; that is, as not symbolic ? " *

Jung's views on this point seem to me far more satisfactory than Freud's. Every element in the dream symbolism ought to receive special interpretation since the " background of the mind " is never the same in any two individuals. What a symbol means for one it may not mean for another, and this must apply to all symbols, since to treat some as possessing a constancy of meaning and others as having a wide variety of meaning would be quite an arbitrary procedure. Moreover, to regard some symbols as always possessing a sexual significance is, it seems to me, rather dangerous. It means that we run the risk of reading into the dream what may not actually be there. Indeed, Freud's contention that all dream interpretation when adequately carried out is found to contain sexual material as its basal elements is attended with this danger. The more obvious interpretations are frequently discarded for others that may be uncon-

* *Analytical Psychology*, p. 301.

sciously suggested by the analyst, or, in the case of auto-analysis, interpretation may be unduly influenced by auto-suggestion. In Jung's method risk of this kind is not nearly so great. It is, therefore, to be preferred to Freud's method even though, perhaps, it could be said of it that it opens the way far too much to freedom of speculation.

Also in its practical value it may be said that Jung's theory is to be preferred to that of Freud. Jung and his school are always asking what is to be gained by the reductive interpretation of dreams. Still I think there is more practical value in the Freudian method than Jung will allow. The main aim of Freudians in dream-analysis is to get at forgotten experiences and repressed impulses. In so far as this aim is realised a better knowledge of oneself results ; and this has proved to be of immense practical value to both the neurotic and the healthy. At the same time, Jung's method is more practical than Freud's. In the unconscious contents as symbolised in the dream are to be found "undifferentiated thoughts and feelings," which give the clue to the better adjustments of the individual to life. Freud's task is finished when he cures the patient of his trouble. The future moral history of the patient does not concern him. Jung feels his work is not finished until he puts the patient on a higher moral plane. For this reason the followers of Freud are always pouring scorn on Jung's theory as being inspired by certain preconceived "mystical" and religious motives, and as being, on this account, "unscientific." The present writer can not understand the application of the epithet "unscientific" to Jung's theory, because in it may be detected a certain "mystical" or "religious" colouring. Neither of these terms need necessarily imply what is unscientific : and, moreover, when the theory of Jung receives impartial consideration it is found to adhere quite as strictly to facts as does Freud's theory. His collective unconscious we reject, not because it does not explain the facts, but because the facts may be otherwise more adequately explained, while his constructive method of interpreting the unconscious is not put forth to supplant, but rather to supplement the Freudian method. In so far as he accepts the views of Freud his position cannot be called unscientific ; in so far as he goes beyond it he is only attributing to the unconscious certain qualities of a prospective or teleological nature, which are already recognised as characteristics of consciousness.

(iii) The Theory of Rivers—

A somewhat different point of view is presented by Dr Rivers in his work, *Instinct and the Unconscious*. Considerations of space limit our discussion to the main features of his theory.

In his contribution to a *Symposium* on *Instinct and the Unconscious*,* in which he advocates the theory that the unconscious consists of repressed instincts, and that the distinguishing mark of instinct as compared with intelligence is " the all or none " principle (we shall presently explain the meaning of this principle), Rivers gives us the following statement : " The early forms of the ' all or none ' reaction, together with the experiences associated with them are incompatible with the graduated reactions which develop later and are dealt with by using a process which . . . has always been closely associated with instinct. I refer to the process of repression or dissociation by which the disturbing experience is not abolished, but becomes separated from the mass of conscious experience which is readily capable of recall. The view I put forward is that this suppressed or dissociated experience makes up the unconscious. . . . The view I have put forward implies a radical difference between the two kinds of reaction with which I deal. Instinctive reactions with

* *Published in British Journal of Psychology*, Vol. X., pp. 5, 6.

their associated experience are thrust into the unconscious because they differ so greatly in nature from those developed later that the two are incompatible with one another and can only be dealt with by the drastic method of suppression. If we consider the development of mind in the light of the view here put forward there is suggested a history in which mental development proceeded for a time along the path of the ' all or none ' reaction. When this path had led the animal kingdom a certain distance in the line of progress a new development began on different lines. The view I put forward is that nature did not proceed simply by modifying the earlier process by graduating its reactions to the needs which the animal had to meet, but started on a new path, developing a new mechanism which utilised such portions of the old as suited its purpose and treated the rest by the process of suppression. In this process those parts of the older form of reaction which were useless or noxious were shut off from the newly developed forms of conscious reaction, only to emerge in sleep or in such states as hypnotism in which the later-developed and controlling influences are in abeyance, or have been replaced by influences of another kind. The suppression, however, is rarely complete, and is always liable to break down under excessive shocks and strains. The fears or phobias and many other, more or less, morbid features of the mental life of man are the expression in indirect and veiled form of this incompleteness of suppression, while the functional nervous disorders and insanities which occur under the stress of adverse circumstances are due to the weakening of the controlling forces and consequent emergence into activity of instinctive reactions which in health are suppressed."

Here we have in summary form the important elements in Rivers' theory. Some explanatory remarks seem necessary to begin with.

(*a*) Reference was made at the beginning of the quotation to the " all or none " principle by which Rivers seeks to distinguish instinct from intelligence. What is the meaning of this principle ? We will give the answer in our author's own words : " An animal or child exposed to danger, which is so recognised as danger that it produces a reaction gives itself to the reaction fully. If it runs away, it runs with every particle of the energy it is capable of putting forth ; if it screams it does so with all the vigour at its command. Its reaction by flight or scream is the same whether the danger be small or great." *

Intelligence which represents a later stage in mental evolution is characterised—in opposition to this principle—by a certain " gradation " of reaction to the nature of the stimuli.

Since the *Symposium* was written Dr Rivers has seen the need of modifying his views on the distinguishing features of instinct. He has come to the conclusion that the " all or none " principle is not applicable to all types of instinctive behaviour and that, therefore, it is not a satisfactory way of distinguishing instinct from intelligence. Accordingly, in his recent work, *Instinct and the Unconscious,* he inclines to the view that instinct must be regarded as an innate mental process, and that the " all or none " principle may be used to distinguish one group of instincts from another. The instincts that are connected with the needs of the individual partake of the " all or none " form. This is true especially of the danger-instincts. Those instincts, on the other hand, that are more closely connected with the needs of the herd are characterised by a gradation of reaction to stimuli, and a fine adjustment of means to ends.

(*b*) The sense in which Dr Rivers uses the word " suppression " differs from its significance in psycho-

* *British Journal of Psychology*, Vol. X., p. 3.

analytic literature. The term has usually been employed by Freud and his followers to denote the conscious process of expulsion of ideas and feelings from the mind, the home of such suppressed material being the fore-conscious. Rivers, however, employs the word in the same sense as the Freudian " repression." He gives no adequate reason for substituting the word " suppression " for " repression," and inasmuch as the latter expression is now well established to signify the process by which what is repugnant to consciousness is rejected, he is not justified in departing from this usage. One result is inevitable, viz., confusion in the minds of readers.

(c) It is necessary to explain a little more explicitly than the quotation does the fact that for Dr Rivers the material of the unconscious consists of instincts and experiences associated with them. It is the earlier, cruder instincts—those characterised by the " all or none " principle—of which the unconscious is formed. These have been repressed (we shall continue to use this term in the Freudian sense—Dr Rivers' suppression), because they are incompatible with later forms of mental reaction.

M⁰Dougall, in his contribution to the *Symposium* from which we have taken the quotation with which we are dealing, rightly asks : what does Dr Rivers mean by the repression of instincts ? Are instincts, as a matter of fact, repressed ? If so, what instincts ? Dr Rivers deals only with the instincts of self-preservation, and with only one group of these, the danger instincts. It is these in repressed form that furnish the material of the unconscious. Dr M⁰Dougall, however, points out that " these instincts continue to determine behaviour of appropriate kinds accompanied by the appropriate emotional experience and, therefore, are not dissociated. The instinctive reaction of running away is not dissociated. He mentions only one other reaction—

screaming in the presence of danger. This is the natural expression of fear and is, therefore, not dissociated." *

Dr Rivers certainly leaves himself open, in the symposium, to this kind of criticism. He does not sufficiently explain what instincts are repressed and how repression of instincts is brought about. In his recent work, however, his theory is amplified ; what is implicit and obscure is made more explicit and clear. He makes use of McDougall's own psychology for his purpose. Closely connected with every instinct is a specific emotion. When danger, for example, threatens the existence or well-being of the individual any one of five different types of reaction may take place—flight, aggression, manipulative activity, immobility, or collapse. With each of these there is connected a specific emotion. Thus, with flight there is associated the emotion of fear, with aggression that of anger, and with collapse, extreme terror. But in the other two types of reaction there is an absence of emotion. Manipulative activity to escape danger must take place without affect. The man who in this way is seeking safety must be cool and collected. Hence all emotion must be repressed. That such repression takes place is proved by the dreams that may follow in which emotion is present often in an intense form.

The same is true, perhaps to a greater degree, of the instinctive reaction of immobility. If immobility is to be a successful way of escape from danger it is clear that it must be absolutely complete. The slightest movement would be of the greatest danger to the person concerned. Such complete immobility can only be brought about by a repression of all affect. This seems quite clear and represents what, as a matter of fact, often happens.

What is actually repressed, then, is not instinct itself,

* *British Journal of Psychology,* Vol. X., p. 40.

but the emotional accompaniment of instinct. On this point Dr Rivers might well be much clearer than he is. He often speaks of what is repressed as instinctive reactions. When we adopt one mode of reacting to danger we thereby repress the others. I don't think this follows at all. In any single situation only one type of reaction can take place at the time, but because we adopt one form of reaction it does not follow that the others are repressed ; any one of them can become the reaction adopted when the next danger situation arises.

What Dr Rivers must have in mind, when he speaks of the unconscious as consisting in repressed instinctive reactions, is the affective accompaniment of the reactions. This is true, not of all instincts, but only of those the primary aim of which is the preservation of the individual. Even within this group of instincts Dr Rivers dwells only on the danger instincts. We are not told whether the unconscious is formed out of the repressed affects of all the instincts of self-preservation or only of the danger instincts, but we conclude that since he deals only with these latter the unconscious, as a matter of fact, is reduced to the repressed emotions connected with some of the instinctive reactions to danger.

What are the general points of agreement between this theory and that of Freud ?

In the first place, it is quite clear that he accepts the general principle of repression though he uses the term suppression instead, and with Freud he regards the experiences that have been repressed in early life as of the greatest importance. Throughout his book he makes great use of a case of claustrophobia that came within his own notice. The case is that of a man who suffered periodically through life from the fear of enclosed spaces. This fear became especially active during his military experiences in a dug-out. The fear

L

of the enclosed space often drove him to pass the night in the open trenches, until finally collapse came and he had to be removed to hospital. He received treatment of various kinds, but with little success until he came under the care of Dr Rivers. The psychoanalytic method was resorted to and after several sittings the trouble was traced back to an emotional experience through which he passed when four years of age. He had been in a dark enclosure alone, when a strange dog appeared and began to growl at him so that he became terror-stricken. Throughout all the years this experience had been forgotten until during psycho-analytic treatment it was brought back to his mind. With the recollection of the incident the old state of terror returned and gradually afterwards there took place relief and improvement.

This incident illustrates the agreement of Freud and Rivers not only on the importance of repression, but more particularly on the importance of the repression of early emotional experiences.

Both writers also agree as to the continued actions in harmful ways of the buried material. In the case of claustrophobia the early experience in its repressed state caused trouble through all the intervening years until the psycho-analytic treatment took place. Again, Dr Rivers recognises that repression is due to conflict or incompatibility between certain natural tendencies and the standards of social life. War neuroses, he says, are often brought about by a conflict between the instinctive reactions to danger, with their emotional accompaniment of fear, and the standard of social life according to which fear is regarded as disgraceful. There is, therefore, a general agreement between Freud and Rivers not only as to the rôle of conflict in the production of the neuroses, but as to the meaning of the conflict. Dr Jones, in a paper in the *British Journal of Psychology* on " Why is the Unconscious Unconscious ? ", admits a general correlation of instinct with the unconscious and of intelligence with consciousness.

The differences, however, between these two writers on the unconscious is far more important than the points of agreement. We shall now indicate two respects in which the differences are radical.

1. The rôle of sex to which Freud attaches the greatest importance is regarded by Rivers as of secondary importance. Thus he says : " According to Freud sexual motives form the predominant elements in the experience which is manifested in the dream . . . There is no doubt that he has overrated the frequency with which sexual elements enter into the production of the dream. Freud himself has provided us with abundant evidence that dreams may depend on such motives as professional jealousy, self-reproaches concerning patients, and other affective states incident upon the life and work of a physician." * When dealing with the neuroses of war in his recent book Dr Rivers goes further and denies altogether the influence of sexual factors in their production. He tells us, for example, that " we now have abundant evidence that those forms of paralysis and contracture, phobia and obsession, which are regarded by Freud and his disciples as pre-eminently the result of suppressed sexual tendencies, occur freely in persons whose sexual life seems to be wholly normal and commonplace, who seem to have been unusually free from those sexual repressions which are so frequent in modern civilisation. It is, of course, obvious that the evidence in this direction, being negative, cannot be conclusive. The point is that while we have over and over again abundant evidence that pathological nervous and mental states are due, it would seem directly, to the strain and shocks of warfare, there is, in my experience, singularly little evidence to show that even indirectly

* *Dreams and Primitive Culture*, p. 9.

and as a subsidiary factor, any part has been taken in the process of causation of conflicts arising out of the activity of suppressed sexual complexes." *

Freudians would argue as against this position that the analyses carried out by Dr Rivers have not been sufficiently thorough, and that if he went deep enough into the ætiological factors of war neuroses he would discover sexual elements at work. Dr Rivers tells us that the pathology of war neuroses is a simple and easily solved matter. He speaks of " the simplicity of the conditions upon which they depend." Freud, however, takes an opposite view. He argues that familiarity with the workings of the unconscious is not to be obtained except by a painful overcoming of the internal obstacles in the way. He regards the problems of even war neuroses as much more obscure and complex than Rivers' theory would admit. They are not the result of painful emotional experiences alone ; these only serve as the proximate cause or occasion of the neuroses and supply the form in which the real trouble manifests itself.

Between these views it is not always easy to decide. Freudians appeal finally to the practical test. In the analyses carried out by them they always come upon some sexual elements at the root of the neurosis, and when these are revealed to the patient relief follows. Rivers, however, appeals to the same test. He tells us that in the cases examined by him there is little evidence that " even indirectly and as a subsidiary factor, any part has been taken in the process of causation by conflicts arising out of the activity of suppressed sexual complexes." In a further work of Dr Rivers, just published,† there is not the least departure from the position here adopted.

Our own opinion coincides in the main with that of

* *Instinct and the Unconscious*, p. 165.
† *Conflict and Dream.*

164

THE UNCONSCIOUS AND PSYCHO-ANALYSIS

Dr Rivers. While admitting the part played by repressed sexual tendencies in the development of mental trouble, we deny that these are always the real cause of the neurosis. As already suggested, it is unwise to approach a patient with the idea that somehow the ætiology in the case must conform to Freud's principles. We are likely, then, to read into the case incorrect interpretations of symbols, and indeed the procedure tends to become far too arbitrary. But we have been led to this conclusion chiefly by a consideration of some cases in connection with which the Freudian principles have been put to the test.

Let us describe a case which we have recently attempted to analyse with a large measure of success, and which has led us to the conclusion we have just expressed.

The patient, Miss A, is about thirty years of age. She admits that she has always been of a highly sensitive disposition. From the age of seven she has been subject to periodical fits of depression and nervous exhaustion. She is of an hysterical disposition, and for many years the fear of nervous collapse has never been absent from her. She is extremely intelligent, as are also the members of her family. Her intelligence made it easy to carry out an analysis of her symptoms, for she was able to grasp the general principles of the Freudian psychology without difficulty.

Altogether six weekly sittings took place. These varied from thirty minutes to an hour each time. At first the patient was asked to describe her feelings and give as clear an account as possible of the history of her trouble. She stated that she was always extremely nervous, but that her tendency to nervous collapse began when she was between seven and eight years of age. At the age of about fourteen her first real breakdown took place. She declares that at this time she did nothing but cry for days. During a visit of the doctor on this occasion she overheard him say to her mother that she would be always subject to nervous collapse, and this greatly troubled her, making her condition much worse. With rest and change she gradually improved, but at intervals the trouble returned. Three years ago, while away from home in England, she broke down completely and a nurse had to be procured to accompany her home. The doctors at this time had grave fears that she would not reach home alive. However, after complete rest and medical treatment she again improved. Since then, no very serious breakdown has taken place, but this is due, she says, to special precaution and care. When the fears of collapse come upon her she decides to have a change and by sheer effort of will she has been able to ward off the trouble.

After learning these facts the principles of psychoanalysis were explained to the patient, and she decided to receive such treatment and advice as an amateur could give.

The writer suggested that she should think over the sort of situations that usually tended most to produce her fears, and to think especially of the events that preceded her first breakdown. At the next sitting she told the following story : One day, when twelve years of age, she was alone in the home with her grandmother. Suddenly the latter took a weak turn and lay down to rest. In a few moments she told the patient that she felt herself weaker and was about to die. She took the patient by the hand, and passed away almost immediately. Miss A remained perfectly calm throughout the whole scene, but a few days afterwards reaction set in, and the first real nervous breakdown took place in which she spent days crying, lost her appetite, and found herself unable to walk.

This event could not be the real cause of her trouble, because the tendency to fear and depression was already present for years previously. At the same time, it cast important light on the nature of the experience that was later discovered as the probable root of her trouble. The presumption was that the real cause of the malady was an analogous experience to that just described. This was confirmed at the next sitting when the patient disclosed the fact that she always has a peculiar dread of death, and that anything that suggested death leads immediately to intense mental depression and fear. The sight of a funeral or cemetery, the scent of certain flowers, or any appearance of suffering in others, always affects her, and in such circumstances sheer determination, in which she has disciplined herself, alone prevents collapse.

The last sitting revealed the experience that, as it seems to me, lay at the root of the trouble. When the patient was between six and seven years of age her sister died, and the circumstances in which the fact became known to her are related in her own words as follows : " One morning on wakening up I was suddenly conscious of an unusual stillness over the house, and on getting frightened I immediately jumped out of bed and ran into the next room to my mother, and on reaching her side the first thing that met my gaze was the dead form of my sister. There were two pennies on her eyes to keep them closed, and I received an intense shock because I thought her eyes were out. I wept passionately for a while and fits of weeping returned at intervals for some time afterwards, but I was so young that I had not the sense to know what was wrong with me."

That this experience was the real cause of Miss A's illness seems clear from the following considerations : (a) It was related with intense emotional accompaniment which showed that for her it was especially significant. (b) Every object that tended most to arouse her fears was associated with this death scene.

Especially significant is the fact that the flowers—the scent of which always created for her a strange dread—turned out to be the same as those out of which wreaths were made for her sister's funeral.

(c) This experience she had largely succeeded in banishing from her mind. She confessed when the memory of it was about to return she always tried to repress it. It is true that the experience was not wholly absent from consciousness ; but the fact that she did not relate this—the most significant experience of her life—until by the method of free association it was brought to the focus of consciousness, shows that she had been repressing it. It does not matter that the experience as a whole was not fully repressed, since, as we have often explained, it is the emotional accompaniment of any experience rather than the experience itself which when repressed produces trouble in the life. It was evidently so in this case.

(d) The results of the treatment bear out the truth of the analysis. It is now twelve months since the analysis was concluded, and the present state of the patient points in the direction of complete cure. She declares that for the first time since she was seven years of age she has not been troubled by the dread of nervous collapse and enjoys a " sense of freedom " hitherto unknown. She is continuing to improve in health.

We do not forget that there are other factors to be taken into account, as well as the emotional shock ; for quite as painful experiences come to most people in the course of life without yielding any such serious results. Two things in this particular case have to be kept in view. First, the experience took place in the early, impressionable years of life, and, secondly, the patient describes herself as having always been of a nervous temperament. If an indirect or subsidiary factor in the case is needed to explain the trouble, then

THE UNCONSCIOUS AND PSYCHO-ANALYSIS

we have it in this inborn nervous characteristic, this predisposition to fear. Dr Sidis has recently expressed the opinion that the phobias described in psychoanalytic literature are modifications of the general predisposition to fear which we all inherit from primitive times. Through the individual experiences of life these predispositions to " fear " become translated into actual " fears," and so we have cases of claustrophobia, agoraphobia, etc. Possibly, however, the inherited predisposition to fear is not so strong as may be supposed. May not the general nervousness and sensitiveness, characteristic of those who later fall victims to mental illness, be due to unwise teaching, and especially to the relating of too many weird ghost stories, all too common in the nursery book ?

However this may be, it is the emotional shock that is at least sometimes the root of the trouble. We are, therefore, in agreement with Dr Rivers that any forgotten painful experience may be the primary factor in the causation of neuroses, and that it is not necessary to go beyond this in search for other factors. In his *Conflict and Dream* this position receives further support, for as against Freud's theory that the dream is the fulfilment of a wish, Dr Rivers maintains that it is rather the expression of a conflict between a number of wishes, or even fears, and the conflict so expressed is not to be traced back to experiences in the early life of the dreamer. His work in war time brought him into touch with men whose dreams could be more reasonably interpreted as expressing quite recent conflicts. He would go so far as to agree with Freud that the symbols of dreams may be traced to " processes characteristic of childhood and youth, which come into activity in sleep." Thus he holds that a dream may be infantile in its imagery without being infantile in its content.

2. The second important distinction between the

169

theories of Rivers and Freud is that the former adheres to the principle of utilitarianism, the latter to that of hedonism. The unconscious for Freud consists of material too painful for conscious thought. For Rivers, on the other hand, the unconscious consists of those elements and processes that are no longer of use to the individual. Freud's theory is more purely psychological than that of Rivers, the latter's being distinctly biological. In the introduction to *Instinct and the Unconscious* Dr Rivers tells us that his aim is to " give a biological account of the psycho-neuroses." *
It is to be expected, therefore, that he should make more of the utilitarian than of the pleasure principle in explaining the nature of the unconscious. His theory is that the very existence of the unconscious depends on the incompatibility between the earlier and later products of evolution. In its early stages of development mental processes are primarily instinctive, and the crude instinctive reactions characterising life at this level are governed by the " all or none " principle. But this type of reaction often clashes with the highest interests of life at its more highly evolved and rational levels, and for this reason they are repressed into the unconscious. The unconscious is formed out of instinctive reactions and experiences associated with them, that are harmful to the organism in its more highly evolved state.

In an interesting way Dr Rivers illustrates his position, (*a*) from those metamorphoses that are common amongst lower forms of life ; (*b*) from certain recent physiological discoveries.

The development of the grub into the butterfly involves two sets of very different experiences. At the caterpillar stage one set of memories connected with its life at this level is needed ; while experiences and, therefore, memories of an entirely different kind belong

* *Conflict and Dream*, p. 1.

to the later stage when the caterpillar has become changed into the butterfly. It would be extremely detrimental to the butterfly if the memories and experiences connected with the caterpillar stage of its existence should come crowding into its life when it has ceased to be a caterpillar. These memories would not only be useless to its new type of existence, but would be positively harmful. Hence the memories of the caterpillar are repressed and dissociated because of their incompatibility with the needs of the butterfly.

All this is to be taken as an analogy of what happens in human life. Cruder types of reaction, which belonged to life when it was swayed by instinct alone, are repressed and dissociated from the higher intellectual processes, because such reactions would be detrimental to the individual.

The second illustration is taken from the work of Head and his colleagues in connection with the construction of the nervous system. It has been discovered from these investigations that there are two different constituents of the afferent side of the nervous system. The one known as the " protopathic " represents the early crude form of reaction to stimulus. With it instincts governed by the " all or none " principle are correlated. The other constituents called " epicritic " represent the later types of behaviour with which intelligence is correlated. In the course of development of the race the protopathic have been superseded by the epicritic and are in a state of repression and dissociation. The epicritic types of reaction are characterised by a greater discriminativeness and gradation. For this reason, as being more useful to the organism, they have been developed and preserved.

The entire theory, then, of Dr Rivers is built on an evolutionary basis. It gives a biological account of the unconscious, and introduces in its support, and as parallels to it, considerations of a physiological kind.

Freud's theory is more consistently psychological. He introduces no physiological archetypes of unconscious processes. The precursors of the unconscious and the conscious which he introduces are mental systems, not physiological correlates.

We may conclude by pointing out how difficult it is, on the principle of utilitarianism adopted by Dr Rivers, to account for all cases of repression. It is, according to him, to the advantage of the individual that repression should take place. But apparently some cases of repression are detrimental to the welfare of the individual. I am not clear how on Dr Rivers' theory he can ultimately explain his own case of claustrophobia. Surely the repression of the early emotional experiences had a harmful effect upon the life. The method of healing adopted by Dr Rivers in which he sought to bring the repressed affect back to full consciousness is the proof of this.

In general, Dr Rivers has to be criticised for his lack of precision in defining the unconscious. In telling us what the unconscious is he depends largely on a method of exclusion, by stating what he does *not* mean by the unconscious. Then he presents us with incidents and illustrations which indicate the existence of the unconscious. But the only approximation to an actual definition is the account of the unconscious as consisting in " instinctive reactions and experiences associated with them." We have seen the difficulty of understanding how instinctive reactions can be unconscious, and have suggested that in the end Dr Rivers intends the unconscious to consist in the emotional accompaniments of some instinctive reactions. As for " experiences associated with them," we hold that experiences do not exist in the unconscious, but rather the traces which experiences leave behind. We shall seek to deal more fully with this definition of the unconscious in the conclusion to which we now turn.

CHAPTER V

CONCLUSION

WE have considered in the foregoing chapters the most important theories of the unconscious. Five groups of these have been distinguished. According to their measure of importance some have received more exhaustive treatment than others. The early theories, which are dealt with in the first chapter, are bound up with the general philosophical systems of their authors, and so share in the strength or weakness of these systems. The four remaining groups constituting the modern theories have been built up on the basis of experimental psychology. Of these the first which we considered, that of Myers, arose out of the study of "psychical phenomena" and was designed especially to explain the nature and origin of these. We suggested that, in the psycho-analytic theories, the phenomena which Myers sought to elucidate were likely to receive a more adequate and natural explanation. The second group of the modern theories, which we called "The Theories of the Subconscious," have much in common with the theories underlying psycho-analysis, the most important of all the theories. Both groups arose in connection with the study of mental disease in its various forms. The psycho-analytic theories, however, are, as we pointed out, much more thorough than the "Subconscious Theories." These latter introduce the concept of dissociation to account for hysterical symptoms. The psycho-analytic theories go further and throw light on those principles according to which dissociation itself may be explained. On this account we regard the theory of Freud and his school as the most important of all the theories of the unconscious. It is to be accepted, however, with certain restrictions and modifications.

In the preceding chapter some objections to the theory were considered, and we shall not return to these, but shall rather confine ourselves to a few points of a more general character. In the first place it must be remembered that the unconscious in any form in which it is held is merely an hypothesis. Pfister * argues that we have as much evidence for the actual existence of the unconscious in ourselves as we have for the existence of consciousness in other people, and psycho-analysts generally speak of the unconscious as something capable of demonstration. This is not so. We have no direct knowledge of the unconscious as we have of consciousness. The term " unconscious " is proof of this. That we should introspect or experience the unconscious is surely a contradiction in terms. If this be so, then, the unconscious can only be accepted hypothetically as a principle that introduces coherence and meaning into otherwise obscure phenomena, and it may be fairly claimed for Freud's theory that, in this respect, it has rendered greater service than any alternative theory. But whether its application is always correct, and whether it is always necessary when it is actually put into operation, are points that are very dubious. It has been so successful in elucidating some forms of phenomena that extreme claims have been made for it, and applications of it made that are unwarrantable.

In discussing the early theories we found that they ended in all sorts of extravagant applications, in Hartmann. The extreme claims that this writer made for his theory was one of the leading factors in the reaction from the study of the subject. There are signs that a similar fate may overtake the modern theories, and for a similar reason.

* *The Psycho-Analytic Method.*

CONCLUSION

We have already noticed the extreme claims which psycho-analysts make with regard to the sexual instincts, and with regard to the rôle of repression to which all cases of forgetting are traced. The same is true of the theory of dream formation. *All* dreams, according to Freud, are wish-fulfilments. This view, as we have seen, has of late been seriously criticised by Dr Rivers. There is no doubt that in very many instances Freud's account of dream formation is correct. It was recognised in principle even before Freud's day and expressions of it may be found scattered through general literature. The following is an instance from Dickens : " In the villages taxers and taxed were fast asleep. Dreaming, perhaps, of banquets, as the starved usually do, and of ease and rest, as the driven slave and the yoked ox may, its lean inhabitants slept soundly, and were fed and freed." * It does not follow, however, that we are to interpret all dreams as wish-fulfilments, especially in the narrow sense in which Freud conceives the meaning of wish.

Similarly with the treatment of everyday mistakes and other " symptomatic " acts. Because some mistakes have been explained as " compromise formations " we have no right to generalise to the extent of holding that all are such, and if unconscious attachments to the father or mother are found to be at the root of some instances of neurotic trouble, we are not to rule out the possibility that other factors may sometimes provide the correct ætiology. Let us take the following illustration as typical of the tendency to push the theory to extremes. It is a case illustrating the displacement of original affect upon play, and is recorded in the *International Journal of Psycho-analysis*, Vol. II, p. 430. " The boy is three years old, exceedingly sturdy, active, and aggressive, and must be

* *Tale of Two Cities*, chap. ix.

almost constantly supervised on account of his sur-
prising impulses. Last fall, when his father and
mother went to the country for their yearly decoration
of the family graves, they took the child with them.
In one part of the family lot is a long slab lying horizon-
tally and marking the location of graves of ancient
members of the family. The parents of the child
started to place flowers on this slab. He did not
approve and vigorously threw on it a handful of earth
which he had gathered from a neighbouring newly-
made grave. The boy was scolded, shaken, or slapped
seven or eight times for persisting in this conduct.
Finally, his father had to hold him forcibly while his
mother finished decorating the graves. The child
was very angry, although quiet, on the way home and
seemed to forget the incident by evening.

"The next morning he went out of doors to play. His
mother happened to look out of the window and saw
that he had dragged a long board from the back and
had begun vigorously to pelt the board with one handful of earth after another. Then he carefully brushed
the earth away. After cleaning the board thoroughly
he left the spot with the air of having completed an
important work and ran into another part of the yard
to play. The play represents a satisfied revenge against
his father, probably also a compensation for the attention bestowed by his mother upon the graves and a
final method of getting his own way by symbolic
play."

The second suggestion in the explanation of the case,
viz., that the play represents " a compensation for the
attention bestowed by his mother upon the graves,"
seems to me unnecessary. It may be argued that no
explanation of the incident is needed, and that the boy
might have brought the board and pelted even it if the
cemetery incident had never happened. It is a common
form of play in which a group of boys often indulge in

order to get rid of some of their surplus energy. But if it is to be connected with the experience of the previous day, it is surely a sufficient explanation that the play represents a symbolic way of having revenge against his father, and of having his own way. He has been described as sulky and aggressive and there is no need to go beyond this for the explanation needed. The writer, however, proceeds to introduce other factors. " The dynamics appear to be the following : The Œdipus complex was manifested by a jealousy directed towards the object occupying his mother's attention— the gravestone. The jealousy towards the gravestone was an animistic survival, in that the child endowed the stone with a hostile personality, and expressed his jealousy and hatred by mud-slinging."

This explanation is not only far fetched, but also quite unnecessary, and it is typical of the procedure of many of Freud's disciples in their eagerness to apply the hypothesis as widely as possible. Psycho-analysis indeed has gone a long way towards robbing consciousness of all its value and power and attributing most of our behaviour entirely to the unconscious. Consciousness is conceived as the slave of the unconscious— the latter being all powerful. Freud tells us * that in this discovery man's narcissism—his feeling of self-esteem and importance—has received its greatest blow. The " ego " received a shock of this kind after the Copernican discoveries, the effect of which was to reveal man's insignificance in the light of the mighty vastness of the universe. It received another severe shock in connection with the Darwinian discoveries, when man's kinship with the lower animals was established. But the greatest blow to man's pride is that which the discoveries of psycho-analysis have administered. These discoveries have robbed consciousness of much of its power and prestige so that " the ego is no

* *Introductory Lectures on Psycho-Analysis.*

longer master in its own house." Behaviourists are glad to make use of these Freudian principles in their extreme position—the denial of consciousness altogether. Mr Bertrand Russell, who, while not a strict behaviourist, approaches that position, may be quoted as an example, in the attempt he has recently made to explain away consciousness.* We usually trust to introspection as the chief method by which conscious processes are known. But since we often take our desires and many other conscious states for what they are not, and are thus deceived, this method is rejected and it is argued that the only way in which knowledge of mental states—if there are such states — can be attained, is by a consideration of behaviour.

To this the reply seems obvious that we can be as easily deceived in observing behaviour as in observing states of consciousness. We may take behaviour for what it is not. Further, if occasionally the verdicts of consciousness turn out to be wrong we are not to argue that it is always so, and there is another point— the fact that people are often mistaken as to what they desire and think does not necessarily discredit consciousness. These conscious states, even though we did not understand their motivation, were for us real at the time.

The fact is that no matter how numerous the arguments of psycho-analysts may be, or how strong the logic of Behaviourists against the power and reality of consciousness we simply cannot deny its importance. Those who do so perhaps do not always understand how near they are to rendering invalid their own theories. Psycho-analysts speak generally of the rationalising power of consciousness as if this were its only function—it works up according to its own demands the thoughts, feelings or strivings that are provided by the unconscious. But surely consciousness

* *Analysis of Mind*, chap. i.

178

does more than rationalise. It reasons and feels and wills and can do so independently of the influences and motives of the unconscious, otherwise what are we to make of psycho-analysis itself ? Either it must come from the unconscious and so is worth no more than our religious concepts which, according to psycho-analysts, are wholly explained as unconscious projections, or else consciousness is capable in itself of the most subtle and independent reasoning, and in every way more important than the unconscious. If the latter alternative is most likely the true one then only those types of behaviour that cannot be explained by consciousness should be referred to the unconscious. The known ought to be applied as widely as possible, but there is the tendency on the part of psycho-analysts to explain even the known by the unknown. For it must be remembered that when we accept the theory of the unconscious to explain otherwise obscure phenomena we are postulating an hypothesis that in itself is very much obscure. But its chief value is that it introduces coherence into a wide variety of phenomena, and enables us to understand their meaning. To these phenomena, however, the principle should be confined.

There is another respect in which the Freudian theory requires for our acceptance, restriction, and modification. We have dealt with its *application ;* we have now to deal with its *statement ;* we are to ask in what sense we are to conceive of the unconscious itself. What is the form of its existence ? Already we have dealt with its material and have advocated the view that it may consist in any tendencies that are subject to repression, and not merely those that are sexual. But in what sense do conscious states that have been inhibited remain in the unconscious ? Freudians find no difficulty in speaking of " unconscious ideas," " unconscious wishes," " unconscious emotions," etc., others, however, find in such a use of language the greatest difficulty. To speak of " the unconscious " is quite intelligible, for this means those states or processes of which, as a matter of fact, we are not conscious. But to suggest that there can be ideas, emotions, wishes, fears, etc., of which we are unconscious sounds contradictory. " Ideas," " emotions " and other such terms imply consciousness, and the phrase " unconscious ideas " amounts, therefore, to " unconscious consciousness."

We have seen that the early theories were brought into disrepute through extravagance in application. But we remember that the second factor that led to a discrediting of these theories was more important. It was the contradictory terms in which the theories were stated. " Unconscious ideas " was an impossible and unthinkable term by which to explain the unconscious. Modifications were suggested, but the reaction towards a purely physiological explanation became complete in Mill and Carpenter.

Precisely the same objection to the modern theories is being raised on every hand. The utmost difficulty is felt by those who demand clearness and consistency of statement in the presentation of unconscious theory, in accepting Freudian terminology ; and the more so because the advocates of the psycho-analytic theory are not content to regard the unconscious as an hypothesis merely, but treat it as reality. Dr Ernest Jones tells us that " unconscious mental processes present all the attributes of mental ones, except that the subject is not aware of them, consciousness thus becomes one attribute of mentality, and not an indispensable one." *

In a recent *Symposium* † strong objection is urged against this view. We shall give two quotations— the first from Mr G. C. Field, the second from Prof. J.

---

* *Papers on Psycho-Analysis*, p. 121.
† *Mind*, Vol. XXXI., p. 413 f.

CONCLUSION

Laird : " When I reflect on what I mean by a wish or an emotion or a feeling I can only find that I know and think of them simply as different forms of consciousness. I cannot find any distinguishable element in these experiences which can be called consciousness, and separated from the other elements even in thought so as to leave anything determinate behind. And to ask us to think of something which has all the characteristics of a wish or a feeling except that it is not conscious seems to me like asking us to think of something which has all the attributes of red or green except that it is not a colour " (p. 414). Prof. Laird quotes Bleuler's definition of the unconscious which coincides with that of Dr Jones and then remarks that " the definition is preposterous. It is like Mr Churchill's cannibals in all respects except the act of devouring the flesh of the victims " (pp. 434-5).

The general reply of psycho-analysts to this type of criticism is that the difficulty is merely due to our habits of thought and speech ; that hitherto we have identified the mental and the conscious ; that this is unwarrantable ; and that if we extend our meaning of the term mental to embrace the unconscious, the difficulty disappears. But this is precisely what cannot be done intelligently unless we regard consciousness as something of no account, as merely accidental and not essential to mental life. Such a view, as Prof. Laird says, " is worse than Epiphenomenalism—what in the world would consciousness be if it had no shreds of character of its own ? " We have thus returned by a different pathway to the point we have already emphasised, viz., psycho-analysis in making so much of the unconscious tends to rob consciousness of all its character and power. There cannot possibly be " unconscious ideas " or " unconscious wishes " unless what introspection reveals to us of our conscious processes is hopelessly astray.

Many attempts have been made so to restate the Freudian theory as to avoid this difficulty, and if it is at all possible to do so, such restatement ought to be attempted.

Some of the attempts to make the theory more intelligible have not been successful. Thus Dr Rivers suggests that instead of speaking of unconscious ideas, wishes, etc., we use the term " unconscious experience." He supports his theory by a reference to the case of claustrophobia, which he makes so much of, and also by an appeal to the principle of heredity, which he says is only another word for " adopted ancestral experience." " If such unconscious elements derived from ancestral experience are by universal assent included within the scope of the mind, it is difficult to understand how it is possible to exclude unconscious experience acquired in the lifetime of the individual." * This is no solution of the problem, for most people will find it quite as difficult to think of " unconscious experience " as of " unconscious ideas," and so far as inherited ancestral experience is concerned we simply deny that we are the subjects of such experience. Something we do inherit, but not experience in the accepted sense of that word. We may speak of the unconscious as the result of experience, but " experiences " is equivalent to " conscious states " and so Rivers' definition of the unconscious leaves us where we were. " It is in every respect identical with consciousness only that awareness is absent."

It may make the difficulty of maintaining this definition clear, if we consider that a conscious state implies an act and an object. If the state is one of cognition then there are always the knowing act and the object known, as well as the knower, to be taken into account. If the state is affective then there are the affect itself and the object which creates it, as well as the subject

* *Instinct and the Unconscious,* p. 161..

of the affective experience to be considered. If the state is conational then both the act of striving or willing together with the end or object of the striving are always involved. What is important in all these mental states is the object. Without the object it is difficult to conceive how the experience could be possible. The object may in itself be another mental act or an image or it may be something material and external. But in either case it is difficult to understand how the object on which the whole mental state depends can be present unconsciously, which it must be if an unconscious state resembles in every way a conscious state except that awareness is absent. Any simple illustration will serve to bring out the impossibility of maintaining in its strictness the Freudian definition of the unconscious. Thus some time ago the writer witnessed the Royal Procession in Belfast. His conscious state at the time, if we consider it cognitively, consisted in an act of perceiving and the object perceived. Feeling, of course, was present, but this also was aroused by the object (the King). Thus the specific conscious state at the moment depended mainly on the object. Sometime afterwards a cinematograph representation of the procession brought the entire experience back again to consciousness. According to the Freudian definition we seem driven to the view that the entire experience must in the meantime have been conserved in the unconscious. But surely this is unthinkable and unnecessary. All that is necessary is that something should have remained in the unconscious, which, when stimulated by the appropriate representation, brought back the memory of the original experience. We may call the thing that persists an impression or a trace or a disposition, and while all these terms are vague and may mean anything within limits, it is clear that we cannot dispense with them unless we advocate the theory of " mnemic causation." Mr Bertrand Russell discusses the advantages of this view for those who wish to maintain a purely psychological account of memory : " You smell peat-smoke and you recall some occasion when you smelt it before. The cause of your recollection so far as hitherto observable phenomena are concerned consists both of the peat-smoke (present stimulus) and of the former occasion (past experience). The same stimulus will not produce the same recollection in another man who did not share your former experience. We cannot, therefore, regard the peat-smoke alone as the cause of your recollection, since it does not have the same effect in other cases. The cause of your recollection must be both the peat-smoke and the past occurrence." *

This theory of " mnemic causation," in which the sole factors essential to the revival of any memory are present stimulus plus past event, is not entirely satisfactory. For it is very difficult to understand how a remote past occurrence together with a present stimulus can be the proximate cause of a present experience. Something else is, or seems to be, necessary, something that is really proximate. Besides, one may ask what is the function of the present stimulus ? What does it stimulate ? It can scarcely be the past occurrence. It must surely be some sort of disposition. Mr Russell sees all this, but rather than admit the possibility of mental dispositions or traces he turns to the doctrine of " engrams," according to which the results of experience become stored in the brain. In this theory he also finds difficulties, and certainly it seems to me that there are quite as many difficulties in the way of holding to the idea that the results of experience consist in brain modifications as there are in the theory of mental traces. We favour the view, therefore, that the unconscious consists of mental dispositions or traces or

* *The Analysis of Mind,* pp. 78, 79.

CONCLUSION

tendencies ; but all these terms are meant to declare our
ignorance of the immediate cause of many of our conscious states rather than any positive assertion of what
the unconscious is.

To leave the question in this form, however, is not to
do justice to the work of Freud. It only brings us to
the position generally held by orthodox psychologists.
Thus Professor Ward in his article on Psychology in the
Encyclopædia Britannica argues that our knowledge
somehow lies stored in the region of the subconscious,
for otherwise it would not be at our disposal when the
need for its recall to consciousness is necessary. " The
name of an author that I have read calls up the slumber-
ing knowledge of the characters and subjects dealt with
in the book. Such bits of knowledge do not exist, as
James held, in the shape of ' vestiges ' on the tissues of
the brain, but rather in the shape of ' presentational '
dispositions."

Professor Stout's views are in close agreement with
those of Professor Ward. In his *Analytical Psychology*,
and *Manual* he expounds the theory that the unconscious
consists of psychical dispositions. " It is impossible to
formulate in words from the introspective standpoint
the most ordinary facts of retentiveness and memory,
without implying that past experiences leave behind
them after their disappearance persistent traces on
which their revival depends." * These traces are not
physiological but psychical. They are left behind by
experience, and out of them the unconscious is built up,
while in turn these dispositions are ever determining
our present states of consciousness.

The views here expressed fairly represent the
treatment which the subject of the unconscious has
hitherto received in general psychology, but in the
" new psychology " much more is included in the
term " unconsciousness " than these writers have

* *Analytical Psychology*, Vol. I., p. 22.

taken account of. This is not to be wondered at, since academic psychology has hitherto confined itself especially to what may be regarded as normal mental functioning, and so the unconscious is discussed mainly in connection with memory, presentations, etc., that is, the orthodox theories only take account of the ideational or cognitive side of the unconscious, and seldom are the emotional or conational factors dealt with. Yet it is in these latter that the essential nature of the unconscious is now supposed to consist. We saw that it is a chief characteristic of Freud's psychology that he drew a clear distinction between the pre-conscious and the unconscious proper. The former stands for the material of the unconscious that can be recalled by the act of attention. In using the terminology suggested we may say that the pre-conscious consists of those traces or dispositions recognised in general psychology, that are capable of being aroused by the appropriate stimuli, and that reveal themselves to consciousness in their true or original character. The unconscious proper consists of those dispositions or tendencies that are not capable of finding their way into consciousness except in disguised forms, until aided by artificial methods. Of these certain distinctions not always recognised ought to be drawn. (1) There are experiences of early life that afterwards powerfully affect behaviour and lead in given situations—times of unusual strain, etc.,—to complete nervous collapse. Dr Rivers' case of claustrophobia is what we have now in mind. But we venture to think that the forgetting of this experience was not due to repression in the Freudian sense. It was forgotten as most experiences are forgotten—or rather never have been retained—that take place in the first few years of life. No special explanation of much of this forgetting seems to be required. It is simply the rule to forget. And an experience of this kind requires special methods

CONCLUSION

—hypnotic, or psycho-analytic—to have them re-called, not because they have been repressed, but because they have occurred so far back in life. It is clear that experiences of an affective nature, such as that which Dr Rivers has made almost classical, taking place at an impressionable age, must leave behind traces or results of some kind that affect later life and behaviour. (2) There are further dispositions or tendencies that are not conscious in the sense that their true charac-ter is not understood. Many of the tendencies included by Freudians in the term unconscious are not themselves unconscious. They are, on the other hand, very conscious. But it is their real meaning that somehow has been kept back from the subject. It is very common, for example, to find a man, not usually regarded as neurotic, yet manifesting all the characteristics of infantile mentality; he hates reality, work is painful, he lacks concentration and is never contented with his present task, he always takes the line of least resistance, and in addition many of those infantile characteristics of a different type are present ; he is completely ego-centric—not only in-considerate of the needs of others, but apparently in-capable of becoming so, characterised by a narcissism of the primary type, in which the libido is almost entirely invested in the self—there is no desire for a love-object beyond himself, no growth even in the ego in the sense in which in the last chapter we saw Freud describes it, consequently no ego-ideal and, therefore, no conscience ; a tendency to remain dirty except when cleanliness to some extent is imposed by social demands, etc. etc.

The foregoing is a general description of a man actu-ally known to me. He is over thirty years of age and the case is typical of very many.

But all these tendencies are not unconscious. What remains unconscious is their meaning. The subject is not aware that they are simply infantile tendencies that he has not been able to outlive. If the subject had explained to him the true nature of such tendencies he would probably be shocked and refuse to admit it. But this is the proof that repression is present somehow. What is repressed, however, is not the tendency but its meaning or true character. It is scarcely an extension of the meaning of the term repression to apply it to what has never been understood, for, according to Freud, the function of this mechanism is not only to thrust from consciousness its objectionable contents, but to prevent the objectionable from ever becoming conscious. It is all the same whether we force from our home the enemy who somehow has gained an entrance or whether prevent him from entering. The only way in which the term as used here may not be in keeping with its strict Freudian use is in applying it to the meaning of tendencies rather than to the tendencies themselves. Such a use of the term, whether it be strictly Freudian or not, is not, I think, without its value. Already we have applied it to a typical case known to us in life. It may also be applied to well-known characters in literature. The reader, for example, of Joseph Le Gras' *Casanova : Adventurer and Lover*, will understand the nature of many of the tendencies which the hero manifests as infantile. He is described as an " unscrupulous egotist," " without morals of any kind," and " he lived apparently without any symptoms of an uneasy conscience." " He clothed himself on each occasion, if he could, with supreme care and according to the very latest fashion. It was the source of continual satisfaction if he strutted about before others ; he paraded equally before his own eyes, and looked at himself in all the mirrors."

In these quotations, (and many others could be included), three well-known infantile character traits are apparent—absence of an ego-ideal, a strong tendency towards exhibitionism, and a pronounced narcissism.

CONCLUSION

In cases such as we have described there is always a twofold danger. In the first place, there is the danger that a man may yield himself entirely to his dominant tendencies, and so become, what many have become, not only indolent and unemployed, but unemployable, or, worse, a debauchee, which Casanova actually did become. Secondly, a conflict may take place between these tendencies and the demands of life which, if it cannot be successfully resolved, may lead to complete mental breakdown. Many of the cases of neurosis described in the literature of psycho-analysis are of this type, and the cure when it takes place consists rather in bringing out the hidden meaning of conscious tendencies than in unearthing unconscious ideas or unconscious tendencies. In this way, also, is explained why it is that an experience of an affective nature to which the analyst traces the troubles of his patient may be revived, and yet the symptoms of the disease may continue. Often indeed the experience is quite open to consciousness and may often be recalled by the patient himself, and yet no relief take place. If cure is effected, as Freud says, by bringing the unconscious into consciousness, then all that can be meant in some cases by this process is getting to understand the meaning of symptoms and tendencies of which we are conscious, and their origin in and connection with past experiences that may also be conscious, or capable of entering consciousness in the ordinary way.

What seems incapable of entering consciousness is the real meaning and nature of these tendencies. But if this is so it is surely wrong to describe the hidden or unknown meaning of a conscious tendency by such terms as " unconscious ideas," " unconscious wishes," and the like. (3) There are, however, facts that point to the actual existence of unconscious tendencies. Apart altogether from the consideration of neurotic symptoms and dreams, from the study of which Freud constructed his theory, it is unquestionably true that under the influence of education, and in response to the demands of civilisation, many of our natural impulses become repressed, and we cease to be conscious of them. The question is, what becomes of these impulses when thrust from consciousness. Already this point has been fully discussed in the preceding chapter. The impulses—whether we define them as libidinal or egoistic or both—pass by sublimation into impulses and activities of a different kind. How sublimation takes place we cannot tell, but that it does so seems to explain the fact that the birth of social or religious impulses often synchronises with the disappearance from consciousness of the " primitive " impulses. This is true whether the processes of the birth of the former and the disappearance of the latter are gradual or sudden.

If this be the case—if the repressed impulses become sublimated—then the question of the unconscious scarcely enters. For the repressed impulses disappear altogether, and others of a different order take their place, not in the unconscious, however, but in consciousness.

Sublimation of repressed psychic material does not, however, always take place, and when it does it is not always complete. It is the impulses that are driven from consciousness and yet have not found an outlet in sublimated activities that form the most important factors of the unconscious; but they exist unconsciously as tendencies or dispositions, not as ideas or wishes. As Mr Bertrand Russell puts it : " The unconscious desire is not something actually existing, but merely a tendency to a certain behaviour — it has exactly the same status as a force in dynamics." *

Such tendencies prove their existence not only in the symptoms of the neurotic and in dreams, but also

* *Analysis of Mind,* p. 38.

in outbursts of passion and types of anti-social conduct such as characterise the behaviour of the mob. Le Bon tells us that one characteristic of crowd psychology, as distinct from individual psychology, is the way in which the unconscious completely dominates the consciousness of the individual as a member of the crowd or mob. So true is this that the individual, when he leaves the mob or when the mob is broken up, can scarcely be brought to admit the crimes with which he is charged. He has been the victim of tendencies, the existence of which in himself he had never suspected. The same tendencies often manifest themselves in the criminal who, not as a member of a mob, but as an individual, commits a crime and afterwards when charged with it declares that he did not know why he committed it, or will protest that he never did commit it. And it is quite conceivable that he is only stating the truth. The tendency that entered consciousness and led to the crime, when again repressed may have carried the memory of the crime with it into unconsciousness. This raises problems for the moralists and the legislators, but we are only concerned at the moment with this question : " Are there unconscious tendencies as well as tendencies the meaning of which is not understood ? " and the facts seem to suggest that there are.

The position at which we have arrived is that the unconscious, as distinct from the preconscious, consists of : (1) the impressions or dispositions left behind by the emotional experiences of early days ; (2) tendencies whose meaning is not recognised or understood ; (3) tendencies that are themselves unconscious, but manifest their presence by " symptomatic " acts and peculiar behaviour.

This account of the unconscious includes more than is admitted in the strict Freudian account according to which the unconscious consists of repressed material and nothing more. We have included in it as well the results of the emotional experiences of early days. These cannot be said to have been repressed, and yet they can only be brought to consciousness by special methods such as psycho-analysis provides. Moreover, we have included in the unconscious the hidden meaning of tendencies that are themselves conscious.

In conclusion, whatever be the fate of the Freudian theory as it now stands, there can be no doubt that Freud's psychology has enabled us to understand and explain life to an extent that was not previously possible. It helps the individual to understand himself better even though he may not carry out any thorough auto-analysis ; it aids him in the solution of his own life's problems ; it prevents him from misunderstanding others ; shows him the meaning of his own prejudices, and in general enables him to adapt himself the better to life. Freud is right when he asks those who pour scorn on psycho-analysis to put it to the test for themselves and they will understand its value. We have found this to be true. Thus in the unanalysed case described in the last chapter, while the man still remains tied to his life of phantasy, and unable to adapt himself to the tasks of life, yet psycho-analysis has not been without some practical results. It has completely changed the attitude of the father from one of harshness to one of sympathy, and has made the relationship between the various members of the home much happier than was previously possible. Thus, in our opinion, the greatest service that the modern study of the unconscious has rendered is that it has furnished us with a new point of view from which to study human life and conduct.

INDEX

INDEX